ABLEISM AS VIOLENCE

Angharad E. Beckett and Miro Griffiths

First published in Great Britain in 2026 by

Policy Press, an imprint of
Bristol University Press
University of Bristol
1-9 Old Park Hill
Bristol
BS2 8BB
UK
t: +44 (0)117 374 6645
e: bup-info@bristol.ac.uk

Details of international sales and distribution partners are available at
policy.bristoluniversitypress.co.uk

DOI: 10.51952/9781447376910

British Library Cataloguing in Publication Data
A catalogue record for this book is available from the British Library

ISBN 978-1-4473-7689-7 hardcover
ISBN 978-1-4473-7690-3 ePub
ISBN 978-1-4473-7691-0 ePDF

Cover design: Lyn Davies
Front cover image: Unsplash/Vasily Kandinsky
Bristol University Press uses environmentally responsible print partners.
Printed and bound by CPI Group (UK) Ltd, Croydon, CR0 4YY

Bristol University Press' authorised representative in the European Union is:
Easy Access System Europe, Mustamäe tee 50, 10621 Tallinn, Estonia,
Email: gpsr.requests@easproject.com

FSC
www.fsc.org
MIX
Paper | Supporting responsible forestry
FSC® C013604

For disabled people and their allies, past and present, whose knowledge and collective resistance exposes ableism as violence, allowing us to imagine more just futures.

Note on cover artwork

We chose the cover artwork by Vasily Kandinsky because its fractured, turbulent energy mirrors the violence of ableism – diffuse, disruptive, and systemic. Its abstraction captures the sense of harm that is everywhere and yet so often unseen.

Contents

Accessible summary vi
Content note xiv
Language note xv
About the authors xvi
Acknowledgements xvii

1 Preamble 1
2 Defining violence and types of violence 4
3 (Re)conceptualising ableism 30
4 From hate crimes to microaggressions 50
5 Confinement: institutions and disabled children/youth 70
6 Assisted dying and terminalism 89
7 Failure of human services during the COVID-19 pandemic 105
8 Not a conclusion 122

References 125
Index 144

Accessible summary

This is an accessible summary of this book.

This summary explains our ideas in clear language. It is designed for:

- People who prefer or need information in a clearer format
- Both disabled and non-disabled readers
- Anyone who wants to understand the main points of the book

Please note: This book discusses serious topics, including discrimination, unfair treatment, and how disabled people can be harmed by society's attitudes and actions. Some people might find these topics upsetting.

About the book

This book is about how disabled people are treated badly by society.

The book is written by Angharad E. Beckett and Miro Griffiths.

Angharad is not disabled. She works as a researcher and has worked with disabled people for many years.

Miro is a disabled person. He uses a powered wheelchair and has personal assistants to help him in his daily life and at work. He works as a government advisor and researcher.

An interesting aspect of this book is the inclusion of conversations between Angharad and Miro. These conversations show how they think about these important topics and share their different experiences.

This book shows how different kinds of harmful treatment – from small everyday insults to serious problems, like the way disabled people were treated during the intense crisis period of COVID-19 – are all connected. Understanding these connections is important.

Chapter 1: Introduction

These are difficult times for disabled people.

Many disabled people face:

- Cuts to benefits or support services
- Barriers to treatment in healthcare
- Being treated as less important than other people

This book explains how society treats disabled people unfairly.

We call this unfair treatment 'ableism as violence'.

This means that when society treats disabled people in ways that harm them – whether physically or in terms of their mental health – such actions are a type of violence.

Violence is not limited to physical assault. It can also involve:

- Ignoring disabled people's needs
- Not giving disabled people proper support
- Making decisions that harm disabled people
- Creating laws that make life harder for disabled people

We aim to help people understand these so we can work toward creating a fairer and more inclusive society.

Chapter 2: What is violence?

When most people think of violence, they think of someone attacking another person physically.

But violence against disabled people happens in many ways.

We describe four types of violence:

1. **Direct violence**: When someone does something harmful to a disabled person.
   - Example: When someone abuses their partner (domestic violence).
   - Example: A support worker roughly handling a disabled person.
2. **Violence by not doing something**: When people don't provide the help that is needed.
   - Example: Not providing ramps for wheelchair users.
   - Example: Not giving proper care in a hospital.
3. **Choosing not to help**: When people in power decide not to give the help they could give, and they are allowed to do this.
   - Example: A doctor deciding not to treat someone because the person has a learning disability.

   o Example: Staff ignoring a disabled person's requests for help.
4. **Taking away support**: When laws or rules remove help that disabled people need.
   o Example: Cutting disability benefits.
   o Example: Removing social care from disabled children or adults.

   These types of violence hurt disabled people's bodies, minds, and lives. They happen because societies often don't value disabled people equally.

Chapter 3: What is ableism?

Ableism is a system that values certain abilities, such as walking, seeing, hearing, communicating or learning in certain ways. It treats people who don't have those abilities as if they are less important or inferior.

Ableism affects many parts of society:

- **Medical care:** Doctors sometimes think lives without certain abilities are not worth living.
- **Buildings:** Many places are designed only for people who can walk or see.
- **Education:** Children who learn differently often get separated from other children.
- **Jobs:** Many employers only want to hire people with certain abilities.
- **Media:** TV shows and films often show disabled people as sad or inspiring rather than as regular people.

Ableism is not just about what individual people think.

It is built into our society through:

- Laws and rules
- How buildings are designed
- How services are organised
- Beliefs about which abilities matter most

Ableism makes violence against disabled people seem normal or acceptable.

It makes people think it's okay to treat people without certain abilities differently or worse.

Chapter 4: Hate crimes and everyday bad treatment

Disabled people often face hate crimes. This is when someone harms a disabled person because they are disabled.

Hate crimes include:

- Physical attacks
- Verbal abuse and threats
- Damage to property
- Harassment

Many hate crimes are not reported because:

- Police don't always recognise them as hate crimes
- Disabled people don't think they will be believed
- Some disabled people can't easily report crimes

Even when hate crimes are reported, they are often not taken seriously.

Everyday bad treatment

Disabled people also face everyday bad treatment that may not be seen as a crime. This includes:

- Being stared at rudely
- Being spoken about, instead of being spoken to directly, for example, when someone says, 'Does she take sugar?'
- Being called 'inspiring' for doing ordinary things
- Not being included in activities
- Being teased or made fun of at school or work

These everyday bad treatments are called 'microaggressions'.

While each incident might be small, they add up over time and can cause stress, anxiety, and make people feel less valued.

Extra risks for some disabled people

Around the world, disabled women and children face even more risk of violence.

Disabled women experience more domestic violence than non-disabled women. Sometimes their partners use their disability against them, like:

- Taking away mobility aids
- Controlling their medication
- Using their need for help to control them

Disabled children are more likely to be abused than non-disabled children. They may:

- Not be believed when they report abuse
- Not know how to tell someone what's happening
- Be separated from other children in special settings
- Not receive the same education about safety and relationships

How disabled people resist

Disabled people fight back against this unfair treatment in many ways. They work together in groups like the *Disability Hate Crime Network* to change how police respond to attacks. Women with disabilities create their own support groups to help each other stay safe. Disabled women also tell their own stories to challenge the idea that they are just victims or inspiration for others.

Chapter 5: When disabled people are kept apart from others

Many disabled people are kept in so-called 'special' places away from the rest of society.

These places include:

- Care homes
- Special residential schools
- Mental health units or hospitals
- Orphanages
- Group homes

Being kept apart from others is harmful in many ways:

- **Loss of freedom:** People can't choose where they live or what they do.
- **Abuse risk:** People in institutions face a higher risk of abuse.
- **Loss of relationships:** It's harder to see family and friends.
- **Loss of skills:** People have fewer chances to learn and develop.

This chapter tells the story of Connor Sparrowhawk. Connor was a young man with learning disabilities and epilepsy. Connor liked buses, music, and recycling. He was a much-loved son and brother.

Connor died in a special unit when he was left alone in a bath. He had a seizure and drowned.

His death could have been prevented with proper care.

Connor's mother, Sara Ryan, has worked hard to get justice for him and other disabled people, so this won't happen to another young person.

Disabled people and families fight against being put in institutions in many ways. Parents refuse when doctors advise them to put their children in institutions. Disabled children in institutions also fight back by refusing orders and making friendships, even though staff call this 'bad behaviour'. These actions challenge the whole system that says some children need to be locked away.

Even smaller, 'home-like' places often have the same problems as big institutions.

They still control disabled people's lives and keep them separate from society.

Moving disabled people into the community is important. But it's not enough if they are still treated unfairly.

Chapter 6: Assisted dying

Assisted dying means helping someone to end their life. It can also mean not giving a person help that will keep them alive.

Miro, one of the authors, is against assisted dying. He works with the *Not Dead Yet* campaign.

The book explains why assisted dying can be dangerous for disabled people:

- It can make disabled lives seem less valuable
- It can be offered instead of proper support
- It can pressure disabled people to choose death
- It can spread to include more and more disabled people, including people who are not going to die soon

In countries with assisted dying:

- It often starts with strict rules
- The rules get less strict over time
- More disabled people become eligible
- Some people choose death because they lack support

The authors worry that assisted dying is becoming a way to deal with social problems like a lack of accessible housing or social care, rather than fixing those problems.

Instead of offering death, society should provide:

- Better healthcare and pain management
- More support services
- Accessible housing
- Financial support
- Community inclusion

The authors believe all lives have value and no one should feel they need to die because they are disabled.

Disabled people work together through groups like *Not Dead Yet* to fight against assisted dying laws. They know from their own experiences how doctors and hospitals already treat disabled lives as being less valuable. They use human rights laws to challenge these policies. They say society should help disabled people to live better lives instead of offering them death.

Chapter 7: What happened during the COVID-19 pandemic

The COVID-19 pandemic showed the unfair treatment of disabled people in society.

In the UK, six out of ten people who died from COVID-19 were disabled.

Disabled people faced:

- **Not getting treatment:** Some doctors decided not to treat disabled people.
    - Some disabled people had Do Not Attempt Resuscitation (DNAR) orders put on them without consent.
    - Some hospitals created rules that made it harder for disabled people to get treatment.
- **Loss of support services:** Many disabled people lost essential support.
    - Support workers couldn't visit
    - Day services closed
    - Therapy sessions stopped
- **Isolation:** Disabled people were left alone.
    - No visitors allowed in care homes
    - No support to use technology to stay connected
    - No checkups from social services
- **Not enough protection:** Disabled people in care homes were not protected.
    - Not enough PPE (masks and gloves)
    - Staff working across multiple homes spreading the virus
    - Not enough testing

The pandemic showed how quickly support for disabled people can disappear in a crisis.

It revealed how society often values disabled lives less than non-disabled lives.

Disabled people helped each other during this period when governments abandoned them. They set up support networks to share food, medicine, and care. They went to court to challenge unfair treatment. They created websites, such as the *COVID-19 Disability Rights Monitor* to document what was really happening when officials ignored their suffering.

Chapter 8: Not a conclusion

This book has shown how society treats disabled people in unfair, hurtful, and sometimes cruel ways.

The authors don't want to call this last chapter a 'conclusion'. This is because the problem of ableism continues to change, and the work to fight it is never finished.

The book can help different people in different ways:

- Researchers can use it to improve their understanding and to identify hidden forms of harm.
- Disability activists can use it to connect different struggles and find better ways to create change.
- Human rights defenders can use it to spot rights violations that might otherwise be missed.

The authors believe that even though ableism is powerful, it is not impossible to change. There are always ways that people can resist and create something different.

Understanding how violence works is the first step toward making change happen.

The authors invite everyone to join them in helping to create a better, inclusive world.

Content note

This book examines violence against disabled people in its many forms. It necessarily contains descriptions of physical and emotional harm, institutional abuse, discriminatory practices, and dehumanising treatments that some readers may find distressing. We have approached these topics with deliberate purpose – not for shock value or voyeuristic effect, but because we believe that confronting uncomfortable realities is necessary for transformation. Much as Boler (2004) argued that pedagogies of discomfort are essential for learning about oppression, we suggest that discussing violence against disabled people requires a willingness to bear witness and sit with difficult knowledge. We walk and wheel a fine line here: highlighting painful realities because they must be known and analysed, while refusing to sensationalise disabled people's suffering. Our aim throughout is to bear witness with care, analyse with rigour, and resist with purpose.

Language note

Throughout this book, we predominantly use identity-first language (for example, 'disabled person' or 'disabled people') rather than person-first language ('person or persons with a disability'), unless directly quoting others. While we respect that many individuals and communities have different preferences regarding disability terminology, our choice reflects our commitment to the social model of disability and the established preferences of the UK disabled people's movement, of which Miro is a member. We recognise that language is political, evolving, and contextual; our usage is not intended to diminish the validity of other approaches but rather to position our work within specific theoretical and activist traditions.

About the authors

Angharad E. Beckett is Professor of Political Sociology and Social Inclusion at the University of Leeds, Affiliate Professor at the University of Malta's Department of Disability Studies, and Fellow of the Academy of Social Sciences. Her research explores disability politics, vulnerability theory, and human rights, with particular focus on disabled children and youth. She is the former Director of the Centre for Disability Studies at Leeds and founder and Editor-in-Chief of the diamond open access *International Journal of Disability and Social Justice*, which reaches readers in over 160 countries. Angharad is also a Fellow of the Royal Society of Arts in recognition of her contribution to social justice and social innovation. Her international standing is reflected in advisory roles with UNICEF and UN committees, and she is currently working with colleagues across four continents. Approaching her work as a non-disabled ally, she practices what she terms 'radical listening' to centre disabled people's expertise and experiences in her scholarship and advocacy.

Miro Griffiths MBE is Associate Professor in Social Policy and Disability Studies at the University of Leeds, where he also serves as Director of the Centre for Disability Studies. As a disabled academic and activist, he brings his lived experience as a wheelchair user with spinal muscular atrophy to his analysis of disability policy and practice. Miro was awarded an MBE in 2015 for his services to disability rights and awareness. His research has focused especially on activism among young disabled people, examining how they navigate independent living challenges and engage with political systems. As a leading member of the *Not Dead Yet UK* campaign and through his work as a government advisor on disability issues, he demonstrates how academic analysis can inform and strengthen advocacy for social justice. His approach combines scholarly rigour with a deep commitment to disability rights that emerges from his experiences in policy development and grassroots organising.

Acknowledgements

We would like to thank everyone at Policy Press who helped bring our vision for this book to fruition.

We extend our sincere appreciation to the anonymous reviewers of our proposal, two of whom have since revealed themselves. We are delighted to thank Professor Beverley Clough (Manchester Metropolitan University) and Dr Lucy Series (Cardiff University) by name for their encouraging support for this book and their precise, constructive feedback.

Dr Lucy Series demonstrated remarkable scholarly generosity by reviewing the complete draft manuscript, as did Dr Kurt Borg of the University of Malta. Both read the manuscript with great care and in the true spirit of critical friendship. This was no small undertaking, and we are deeply grateful to them both.

We remain, of course, fully responsible for the book's contents and arguments. Any errors or omissions are entirely our own.

Finally, we thank our wonderful families and friends for sustaining us through life's challenges and making our days so much more interesting and enjoyable. As one anonymous writer observed, 'Family and friends are the invisible threads that weave the tapestry of our lives'.

1

Preamble

Violence in plain sight

This book is about the visible and invisible forms of violence that shape disabled lives and *leave their mark*. Disabled people live 'in the wake' (Sharpe, 2016) of violence. Violence against disabled people is all around us. It exists in the hospital wards where Do Not Attempt Resuscitation (DNAR) orders are applied without consent. It operates through welfare systems that withdraw vital support and push people into poverty. It manifests in institutional spaces, where restraint is routine and segregation is normalised. It permeates everyday interactions where invalidation chips away at disabled people's sense of self-confidence and worth, ultimately damaging their mental health and wellbeing. During the COVID-19 pandemic, it emerged with brutal clarity when triage protocols systematically deprioritised disabled lives. This violence is not random or exceptional – it is structured, systematic, and sustained through interconnected institutions, discourses, and practices. This systematic violence against disabled people is not only a profound social injustice but also a violation of fundamental human rights. Most obviously, it is a violation of Articles 15 and 16 of the UN Convention on the Rights of Persons with Disabilities (CRPD, 2006), which explicitly require states to protect disabled people from torture, cruelty, and all forms of exploitation, violence, and abuse.

These are dangerous times for disabled people globally, as we confront a mounting polycrisis in which authoritarianism, economic volatility, ecological breakdown, and the full range of oppressions, including ableism, interact in mutually reinforcing and amplifying ways. Hard-won rights are being rolled back, systems of care and protection dismantled, and disabled lives are increasingly treated as expendable. In this context, disabled people face not only exclusion or neglect, but also active devaluation and threats through policy, rhetoric, and the withdrawal of even the most basic of supports.

This treatment of disabled people persists partly because disability issues remain stubbornly marginalised even within broader social justice movements. Disability rights seem to be among the lower priorities in Diversity, Equality and Inclusion (DEI) agendas – the 'poor relation' receiving nominal acknowledgement but rarely substantive commitment. This marginalisation has only intensified in recent years. The rise of right-wing populist movements globally has created an environment where protections for disabled people are increasingly portrayed as unnecessary accommodations rather than fundamental rights.

In early 2025, the UK's supposedly left-wing Labour government proposed reforms to disability and health-related benefits that many commentators argued would revive the austerity logic of 2010–2020, a period already shown to have had devastating effects on disabled people. Following backlash from its own MPs and widespread criticism, the government partially retreated in June 2025. The concessions, however, only protect existing claimants; new applicants will still face reduced entitlements and increased conditionality. The threat to disabled people's welfare therefore remains acute.

Research by Martin et al (2021) found that between 2010 and 2014, in England alone, spending constraints on health and social care were associated with an estimated 57,550 excess deaths. It is against this backdrop that the government's Green Paper proposed abolishing the Work Capability Assessment by 2028. Proposals would also mean losing the crucial 'substantial risk' safeguards that have allowed people at risk of suicide or serious harm to be recognised as not fit for work. Despite acknowledging these risks, the Department for Work and Pensions intends to replace the Work Capability Assessment with a system that imposes 'support conversations' and heightened conditionality for most new claimants, with only a narrow group of people with severe lifelong conditions exempted. For many, the proposed change will mean lower income support and repeated engagement with work-focused processes, even where they are unable to work.

It is against this backdrop that we position our work. We are fired by anger, but determined to channel that anger into rigorous, critical scholarship. We write as an act of resistance.

As scholars with different relationships to disability but a shared commitment to justice, we bring complementary perspectives to our analysis. Angharad writes as a non-disabled person whose career in Disability Studies began through volunteer work with a self-advocacy group for people with learning difficulties – an experience that transformed her understanding of injustice and disabled people's fight for equal citizenship. In her research and advocacy work she seeks to pract*ise* and pract*ice* allyship, acknowledging her privileges and recognising the expertise that comes from disabled people's lived experience. Miro, in addition to his academic expertise in Disability Studies, brings his perspective as a disabled person with spinal muscular atrophy who uses a powered wheelchair and requires 24-hour personal assistance. His background in disability activism, since his teenage years, combined with his role as a government social policy advisor, has established him as an experienced policy operative with deep insights into systemic barriers.

Our approach and the journey ahead

This book deliberately weaves together a more traditional presentation of academic analysis with direct dialogue. Each subsequent chapter includes 'cutaways' – conversational interludes where we step back from formal academic prose to speak directly with each other. These dialogues are not merely illustrative asides; they reveal the dialogic nature of knowledge production. Like filmmakers using cutaway shots to enrich storytelling, we hope these dialogues offer insight into our thinking and our academic activism, showing how theory, practice and personal biographies intertwine in our approach to disability justice.

In Chapter 2, we establish our conceptual framework for understanding violence against disabled people. We expand conventional definitions of violence to capture its full spectrum, developing an original typology with four interconnected forms of violence: commission (direct harmful acts), omission (harm through inaction), commission by omission (deliberate decisions not to act despite having the capacity to do so, enabled by discretionary authority that allows fundamental duties to be treated as conditional), and omission by commission (policies that actively remove protections or withdraw support from disabled people). We examine how international frameworks engage with these forms of violence, revealing both opportunities and tensions in the way violence against disabled people is conceptualised within rights frameworks.

In Chapter 3, we move from typology construction to theorisation, reconceptualising ableism as a '*dispositif* of violence'. Drawing upon the work of Michel Foucault and Gilles Deleuze we map how ableism operates as an assemblage that determines what can be seen, said, and done in relation to disability. We examine how disabled people are subjectivised within these power relations while identifying points of resistance and escape.

The subsequent chapters apply the typology and theoretical framework to various manifestations: interpersonal violence and microaggressions (Chapter 4), confinement (Chapter 5), assisted dying and terminalism (Chapter 6), and the failures of human services during the COVID-19 pandemic (Chapter 7). Our final chapter is not a conclusion but a pause – a reflective moment that resists closure. We recognise that ableism, as a *dispositif* of violence, operates as a dynamic network that continuously reconfigures. Understanding how violence operates is the first step toward imagining something different. Violence is not inevitable. We *can* intervene.

We invite you to join us on this journey – one that will take us through difficult terrain but with purpose and hope.

2

Defining violence and types of violence

> Violence matters. It wrecks lives. It causes injury and misery. Violence is both a cause and consequence of inequality. It is a violation of human rights. Violence is a detriment to health. (Walby et al, 2017, p 1).

To define violence clearly and purposefully matters profoundly. As stated in the opening quotation, it *wrecks lives*. Definitions carry weight, steering our analyses and shaping political, institutional, and social responses. This chapter, and the next, seek to define violence as it relates to disabled people and, critically, to ableism. Our goal is to demonstrate not only that violence against disabled people exists, but that it operates systemically, institutionally, and normatively – intimately woven into structural configurations that devalue certain lives and render them precarious. Central to our analysis is how violence operates through different manipulations of the relationships of duty and responsibility within ableist systems, revealing the sophisticated mechanisms through which harm is produced, legitimised, and sustained.

Our typology

Violence remains a contested concept across disciplines, with definitions varying considerably depending upon theoretical traditions and analytical priorities. We begin by setting forth our position, drawing upon established understandings, while developing our own distinctive approach that foregrounds the operations of duty and discretion within ableist power relations.

The World Health Organization (WHO, 2002, p 5, drawing upon their earlier 1996 definition) offered us a helpful foundation for our approach, defining violence as the 'the intentional use of physical force or power, threatened or actual, against oneself, another person, or against a group or community, that either results in or has a high likelihood of resulting in injury, death, psychological harm, maldevelopment or deprivation'.

This definition includes not only physical force but also 'power' – thus broadening our understanding to encompass 'those acts that result from a power relationship, including threats and intimidation' and, crucially, 'neglect or acts of omission' (WHO, 2002, p 5). This recognition of power relationships and omission proves particularly valuable for understanding violence against disabled people, where harm often operates through the manipulation of care relationships and professional discretion.

Sylvia Walby's 2013 and 2017 work with colleagues also provided a crucial grounding for our conceptualisation. She insists that violence, to be such, must produce measurable, embodied harm – physical or psychological. In this way, she resists expanding its conceptualisation into purely metaphorical or abstract domains. Interestingly, we find in Foucault (1982, p 789) a sentiment close to that of Walby and colleagues: 'A relationship of violence acts upon a body or upon things; it forces, it bends, it breaks on the wheel, it destroys, or it closes the door on all possibilities'.

This grounding in real, experienced harm has provided an essential empirical anchor for our analysis. That said, we disagree with Walby et al's (2017, p 42) argument that violence necessarily involves 'actual, intended or threatened, direct or indirect physical contact'. We recognise that violence against disabled people often operates through the absence of action – various types of omission that manipulate fundamental relationships of duty and responsibility. We also decouple violence from the necessity to involve physical contact. The withdrawal of support, institutional neglect, and systematic deprioritisation of disabled lives may involve no physical contact whatsoever, yet produce profound physical and psychological harm that would meet Walby's own criterion of measurable damage to people's physical and/or psychological wellbeing.

Drawing upon these foundations, we propose a typology comprising four distinct yet interconnected actions. Our framework recognises that understanding violence against disabled people necessarily involves questions of duty and responsibility – not merely formal legal obligations, but the broader web of moral, social, and ethical duties that structure relationships between people and between people and institutions. This web operates across interpersonal levels (the moral and social duties we owe each other in families, communities, and workplaces) and institutional levels (the responsibilities that governments, corporations, schools, and health systems have towards individuals and communities). These encompass everything from basic human obligations, such as not injuring, humiliating, excluding, or abandoning others, to professional responsibilities of care and institutional duties of protection and support. These duties are borne by different actors – individuals in their personal relationships, professionals through their roles and training, institutions through their mandates and policies, and states through their legal obligations – with each level creating overlapping webs of responsibility that ableism systematically manipulates. This approach reveals the sophisticated operations of power that require different analytical and political responses. We identify four distinct yet interconnected mechanisms through which duties to protect, support, or refrain from harming disabled people are violated, avoided, or systematically undermined:

1. **Commission**: When individuals or institutions engage in actions that directly harm disabled people.
2. **Omission**: When individuals or institutions fail to act, leading to serious harm to disabled people.
3. **Commission by omission**: When an individual with power and capacity to protect or support disabled people deliberately chooses not to act, enabled by legal or policy discretion, thus causing harm.
4. **Omission by commission**: When a law or policy actively removes, withdraws, or denies rights or protections from disabled people, explicitly withholding previously available or reasonably expected support, resulting in harm.

We provide a visual representation of this typology in Figure 2.1.

These are, of course, 'constructed types' as explained by McKinney (1966), which we have developed to facilitate description, comparison, and analysis. Importantly, these forms of violence often interconnect in systematic ways. For example, when policies systematically withdraw protections or narrow legal requirements (omission by commission), they create institutional environments where professionals can exercise discretionary authority to deny care or support while claiming to follow policy guidance (commission by omission). The systematic removal of safeguards enables individual

Figure 2.1: Venn diagram of typology of violence

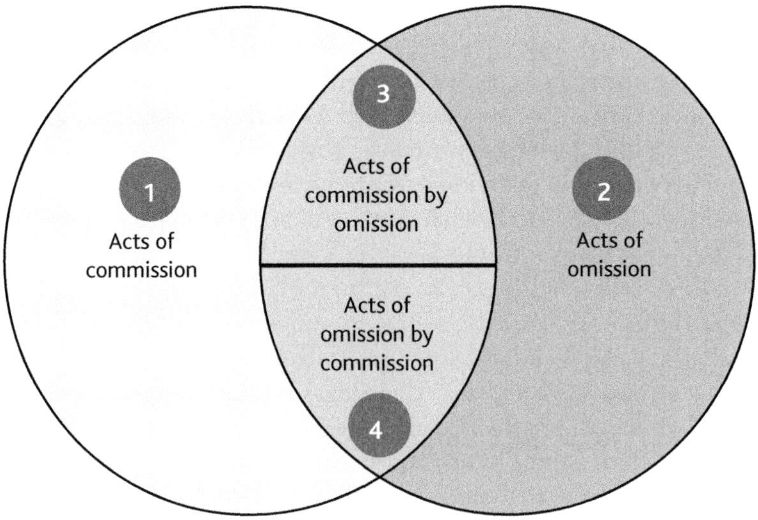

Source: © A.E. Beckett 2026

professionals to make discriminatory choices that would otherwise be recognised as clear violations of duty.

This typology allows us to capture the full spectrum of violence experienced by disabled people – from direct, interpersonal acts to systemic neglect, discretionary denial of support, and formal withdrawal of protection. Each category represents distinct mechanisms through which harm is produced and legitimised, yet all result in measurable damage to disabled people's physical and/or psychological wellbeing. We recognise that empirical cases often blur these boundaries, with the same incident potentially involving multiple forms of violence simultaneously. Our purpose is not taxonomic precision but analytical clarity – revealing how different mechanisms of harm operate and interconnect within the broader *dispositif*. We hope that this heuristic typology will prove useful to others when employed empirically as part of a typological methodology (Winch, 1947).

Making violence concrete: examples in disability contexts

To illustrate how our typology applies specifically to violence against disabled people, we offer concrete examples of each type. These examples demonstrate how different mechanisms of duty-manipulation operate across the interpersonal and institutional levels we have identified, revealing why distinct analytical and political responses are required.

Violence by commission encompasses the most recognisable forms of harm – violations of the fundamental duty not to harm others. It includes hate crimes against disabled people, such as verbal abuse, physical assault, harassment, and, in some cases, murder. It also includes institutional mistreatment, such as forceful restraint in psychiatric facilities or forced sterilisation. These acts produce direct, embodied harm through the active application of force or power. The damage is both immediate and visible; however, its legitimation often comes wrapped in professional authority – hidden behind euphemisms such as 'control', 'management of challenging behaviours' or even 'treatment'. Whether perpetrated by individuals or institutions, these acts represent direct violations of basic obligations not to harm disabled people.

Violence by omission operates through inaction that produces harm – the failure to fulfil duties to act, protect, or provide support when such duties (which can be moral, not just legal) exist. This operates across both interpersonal and institutional levels. Community members failing to act against the persistent bullying of a disabled person reflects broader cultural norms that position disabled people as less deserving of protection and intervention. A building management company failing to maintain a lift or offer alternative, accessible accommodation, leaving a wheelchair user trapped in their apartment, unable to evacuate during a fire. A hospital failing to provide accessible communication methods for a deaf patient, resulting in misdiagnosis or delayed treatment.

These harms result not from direct action but from a failure to act – a failure to provide vital assistance or accommodations. The violence of omission is just as harmful as commission, yet it remains less visible precisely because it operates through absence rather than presence.

Commission by omission involves a deliberate decision by someone who has the capacity to provide protection or support but who also has the discretionary authority *not to act*. This differs from simple omission because it involves the conscious exercise of legitimate power to avoid fulfilling duties, rather than just a failure to act. A doctor legally placing a DNAR order on a patient with learning disabilities through unilateral judgement rather than consultation with the patient or their family, based upon ableist assumptions about that patient's quality of life. Other medical professionals dismissing disabled people's reports of pain, using their clinical authority to reframe genuine medical needs as drug-seeking behaviour or attention-seeking. Child protection workers who have the authority to investigate abuse allegations deciding not to pursue cases involving disabled children based on assumptions that these children will not make credible witnesses. These actions are not passive oversights; rather, they are active choices enabled by discretionary power, which uses professional or institutionally granted authority to hollow out existing duties of care by reinterpreting fundamental obligations as discretionary choices. This transformation shifts the imperative 'must protect' to 'may choose *not to* protect'. This form of violence operates through what might be termed 'purposeful neglect' – using discretionary power to render fundamental duties conditional based on judgements about whose lives merit full consideration and whose accounts can be trusted or believed. It is perhaps the most insidious form of violence because it masquerades as 'reasonable professional practice' while encoding deeply ableist assumptions about the value of disabled lives and the credibility of disabled voices within apparently neutral decision-making processes.

Omission by commission occurs when institutional or legislative actors formally redefine or remove duties of protection and support through policy changes, systematically rewriting the existing obligations. In our typology, this differs from commission by omission because it operates through blanket policy decisions rather than individual discretionary choices. This might include legislation that reduces disability benefits below subsistence levels or policy directives suspending legal requirements to provide reasonable accommodations during emergencies. It could also include the deliberate exclusion of certain categories of disabled people from accessing support services based on cost-benefit analyses. Here, the harm comes from explicit institutional decisions to remove support and deny rights – formally withdrawing previously available or reasonably expected protections. This is violence enacted through policy. It destroys lives, dismantles independence, and, in some cases, results in premature death.

These examples illustrate how our typology captures both the overt and covert forms of violence experienced by disabled people, operating through different manipulations of duty relationships across interpersonal and institutional levels. While hate crimes and forced interventions may be more readily recognised as violence, the failures to act when moral and legal duties exist, discretionary denial of care and protection, and formal blanket withdrawal of support are equally harmful in their effects, producing measurable damage to disabled people's wellbeing, autonomy, and often their very survival. The distinctions between these types matter because they reveal different operations of power that require different analytical and political responses. Individual perpetrators of commission require criminal justice responses. Omission at interpersonal levels calls for cultural change, while those at the institutional level require policy reform, accountability, and external inspection. Discretionary abuse of authority requires, among other interventions, robust scrutiny of discretionary powers and independent review of the application of professional authority, while systematic policy withdrawal requires legislative and political challenge. The value of this typology, we suggest, lies in its ability to name violence where it might otherwise be obscured, sanitised, or reframed as necessary administrative action. By recognising these different mechanisms of harm – and the different manipulations of duty relationships they represent – we can more effectively identify, analyse, and challenge the full spectrum of violence against disabled people.

Further, these categories often operate simultaneously. The Winterbourne View scandal in the UK exemplifies this complexity: staff violence against residents with learning disabilities (commission), regulatory failures to adequately monitor the facility (omission), care quality inspectors choosing not to act on available evidence of harm (commission by omission), and policy decisions that maintained inadequate oversight systems (omission by commission) all functioned together as interconnected elements of systematic abuse.

Why violence against disabled people remains unrecognised

Before examining how violence is recognised, missed, or obscured within legal frameworks, we want to address a thorny question: why is it that societies around the world struggle to recognise violence against disabled people as violence at all? Even the more obvious types, such as hate crimes, are not always recognised. What mechanisms enable this systematic misrecognition?

Several scholars offer complementary analyses to answer this question. Hughes (2012) examines the emotional infrastructure of ableism, identifying fear, pity, and disgust as affective building blocks that sustain violence against disabled people. Shildrick (2002, 2012) demonstrates how ableism stems from deeper existential anxieties about bodily instability and interdependency, disrupting normative fantasies of bodily integrity. Goodley (2014, p 117) describes the 'psychopathology of the normals' that manifests through mechanisms of disavowal, often rationalised through seemingly benevolent practices. Ahmed's (2004) concept of 'affective economies' explains how these emotional responses 'stick' to disabled bodies, producing stigma.

The concept of vulnerability is crucial to understanding these processes of misrecognition. Beckett (2006, 2025) offers a framework that positions vulnerability as both a critical tool and a dangerously misapplied label. She argues that vulnerability has become problematically associated with disabled people, creating a false binary that justifies paternalistic interventions while obscuring the universal nature of human interdependence. She emphasises our universal interdependence on others, environments, and institutions. Importantly, Grech (2015) and Meekosha (2011) remind us that this positioning of disabled people as inherently vulnerable is not universal but largely emerges from Western biomedical traditions exported through colonial contexts. Many indigenous frameworks conceptualise disability and interdependence quite differently.

We suggest that ableist violence remains unrecognised precisely because most societies today refuse to acknowledge this shared precarity – projecting vulnerability onto disabled bodies while maintaining the fiction of non-disabled invulnerability. This projection operates through the manipulation of duty relationships that we have identified. When disabled people are constructed as an inherently vulnerable Other, duties to protect become reframed as benevolent interventions rather than fundamental human-to-human obligations, while duties not to harm become conditional upon professional judgements about capacity and worth. Vulnerability, as a concept, becomes dangerous, as Beckett (2006) noted, when it becomes falsely attached only to certain groups rather than recognised as a universal human condition, *and* when it is misrecognised as solely inherent rather than understanding how social factors also systematically increase vulnerability for some while providing protection for others.

While other explanations exist, the operations of this affective infrastructure convincingly explain why ableist violence remains largely invisible. When embedded cultural anxieties operate through emotional registers that legitimise exclusion, violence transforms into apparently necessary or beneficial action, allowing it to remain unrecognised as violence at all. The sophisticated manipulation of duty relationships – from rendering fundamental obligations conditional, to formally withdrawing protections through policy – becomes naturalised as a 'reasonable' response to inherent vulnerability rather than recognised as systematic harm.

Legal recognition of violence: international frameworks

Having established our typology of violence, we will now examine whether, and if so how, these forms of violence are recognised within international legal frameworks. The law speaks powerfully to what societies value. It codifies which harms are perceived to warrant recognition and redress, establishing formal duties of protection and support. Despite their lofty rhetoric, international frameworks frequently fail to protect disabled people from the very violence they purport to prevent – not merely through implementation failures, but through structural features that enable the manipulation of the duty relationships we have identified. We have chosen to focus on international law for several crucial reasons. First, international frameworks establish shared normative standards that signatories (States) have formally committed to uphold, regardless of their chosen approach to implementation at the national level. Second, these frameworks create a common reference point across different national contexts, providing a baseline against which to measure state failures. Third, States Parties have explicit obligations under these frameworks, making their failures to protect disabled people not only moral but also legal failures – breaches of binding commitments that they have voluntarily undertaken. While a comprehensive cross-national comparison of domestic legal frameworks lies beyond the scope of this book, international law provides a revealing lens through which to examine the recognition, or lack of recognition, of violence against disabled people.

Our analysis draws upon major international human rights instruments, with particular attention to the CRPD as the most significant legal framework specifically addressing the rights of disabled people. We examine how these frameworks explicitly or implicitly recognise the different types of violence in our typology and where significant gaps remain – gaps that are not accidental oversights but structural features of legal systems that remain deeply imbued with ableism and its manipulation of fundamental duty relationships.

The content of Table 2.1 might suggest, at first glance, that international frameworks provide comprehensive protection against violence toward disabled people. Such a conclusion would be profoundly mistaken. The reality on the ground – the lived experience of disabled people worldwide – tells a starkly different story. These frameworks, despite their apparent coverage, have many loopholes, exceptions, and implementation gaps that render their protections largely theoretical. More fundamentally, they often fail to recognise how violence operates through the sophisticated manipulation of duty relationships that our typology reveals.

Consider the case of Michael Hickson, a 46-year-old African American man and quadriplegic, who contracted COVID-19 in 2020. Despite the clear protections enshrined in CRPD Articles 10 (right to life) and 25 (right to health), Mr Hickson was denied admission to intensive care based on a frailty assessment that categorised him as unlikely to benefit from such interventions. His family watched in despair as he was moved to palliative

Table 2.1: International legal frameworks and their recognition of types of violence against disabled people

Framework	Key articles/provisions	Recognition of violence types – an interpretive reading
UN Convention on the Rights of Persons with Disabilities (CRPD)	Article 10: Right to life.	Recognises violence by commission (harmful practices) and violence by omission (denial of care).
	Article 11: Situations of risk and humanitarian emergencies.	Addresses omission by commission (removal of protections during crises) and violence by omission (failure to include disabled people in emergency planning).
	Article 12: Equal recognition before the law.	Identifies commission by omission (discretionary denial of legal capacity leading to harmful practices).
	Article 14: Liberty and security of person.	Addresses violence by commission (institutionalisation) and omission by commission (legal removal of liberty protections).
	Article 15: Freedom from torture or cruel, inhuman, or degrading treatment.	Recognises violence by commission (restraint, seclusion) authorised through omission by commission (permitted exceptions).
	Article 16: Freedom from exploitation, violence, and abuse.	Directly addresses violence by commission while recognising violence by omission (failure to monitor).
	Article 17: Protecting the integrity of the person.	Addresses violence by commission (forced interventions).
	Article 19: Living independently and community inclusion.	Recognises violence by omission (institutional segregation despite community living rights).
	Article 25: Health.	Addresses commission by omission (discretionary denial of care) and violence by omission (inaccessible healthcare).
	Article 28: Adequate standard of living and social protection.	Recognises omission by commission (withdrawal of benefits and supports).
UN Convention Against Torture (CAT)	Articles 2 & 16: Prevention of cruel, inhuman, or degrading treatment.	Addresses violence by commission (institutional practices) with limited recognition of other types.

Table 2.1: International legal frameworks and their recognition of types of violence against disabled people (continued)

Framework	Key articles/provisions	Recognition of violence types – an interpretive reading
UN Convention on the Rights of the Child (CRC)	Article 19: Protection from all forms of violence.	Recognises violence by commission and omission (neglect and failure to monitor) against disabled children with limited attention to other forms.
	Article 23: Rights of disabled children.	Partially addresses violence by omission (failure to provide necessary support).
Convention on the Elimination of All Forms of Discrimination Against Women (CEDAW)	General Recommendation 35: Gender-based violence.	Limited recognition of intersectional violence affecting disabled women.
International Covenant on Economic, Social and Cultural Rights (ICESCR)	Article 2(2): Non-discrimination.	Addresses violence by omission (neglect of disability rights).
	Articles 6 & 7: Right to work.	Recognises violence by omission (economic marginalisation).
	Article 11: Right to an adequate standard of living.	Recognises omission by commission (e.g. austerity measures).
	Article 12: Right to health.	Addresses violence by omission (healthcare neglect) and commission by omission (resource allocation decisions).
WHO Global Disability Action Plan 2014–2021	Objectives on removing barriers and improving access.	Addresses violence by omission (implementation failures).
Sendai Framework for Disaster Risk Reduction (2015–2030)	Inclusion of disabled people in disaster planning.	Recognises violence by omission (neglect in emergency preparedness).

care without their consent. Michael died, becoming one of countless disabled people whose rights under international law were recognised in theory but denied in practice through the discretionary manipulation of clinical duties (Wilson, 2021). We will return to Mr Hickson's case in Chapter 7. While the legal case surrounding his death is pending, for his family and supporters, his death exemplifies commission by omission – medical professionals with discretionary authority rendering fundamental duties of care conditional upon ableist judgements about whose lives merit full protection.

Law as violence: from protection to permission

In addition to the issue of laws that appear to be unenforceable, there is another uncomfortable issue, all too often overlooked: how the law itself can function as a mechanism through which violence against disabled people operates. As Steele (2014) argues in her concept of 'lawful' and 'good' violence, law is not merely a solution to violence but can be implicated in violence itself. Legal frameworks establish the 'contours of lawful violence' – defining which forms of violence are prohibited and which are permitted (Steele, 2014, p 473). For disabled people, these contours often operate differently, creating what she terms a 'differential lawfulness of violence' based on perceived capacity and normality (Steele, 2014, p 475).

We suggest that the Mental Health Units (Use of Force) Act 2018 in the UK (commonly known as 'Seni's Law') represents an example of what Steele describes. This legislation emerged following the death of Olaseni Lewis, a young Black man who died after being restrained by police officers in a mental health unit. He was handcuffed, leg-restrained, and held face down (a form of prone restraint, known to be dangerous). During the restraint, he lost consciousness, but police officers believed him to be feigning, and medical professionals did not intervene. He later died of cerebral hypoxia (lack of oxygen to the brain) on 3 September 2010. While establishing important safeguards, the legislation nevertheless ultimately 'regulates' rather than 'prohibits' the use of force against people in mental health crises. It legitimises certain uses of force that would be unlawful if used against people not labelled as having psychosocial disabilities.

Similarly, restraint provisions in mental capacity legislation explicitly define and permit forms of control that would otherwise constitute assault. Section 6 of the UK Mental Capacity Act 2005, for instance, permits restraint when considered 'necessary' and 'proportionate' to prevent harm to someone deemed to lack capacity. The very existence of such provisions reveals how legal frameworks construct disabled bodies as legitimate targets of force and control. These legal mechanisms operate through all four forms of violence in our typology: commission (direct physical restraint), omission (failing to require alternative responses), commission by omission (legitimising professional judgement to deliberately withhold protections available to non-disabled people), and omission by commission (systematically removing protections through specific legal provisions targeting disabled people).

Mechanisms that obscure ableist violence within legal frameworks

Extending this analysis, we conclude that several mechanisms systematically obscure violence against disabled people within legal frameworks. These function not as accidental flaws but as structural features that maintain the status quo through the organised manipulation of duty relationships.

Exception clauses: Many human rights instruments permit limitations 'in accordance with law' or for 'public health' reasons. Such exceptions create legal justifications that have systematically enabled coercive psychiatric interventions against people with psychosocial disabilities. They appear as neutral safeguards. This connects directly to what Foucault (1998) calls the 'will to knowledge/truth' – a system that presents itself as neutral and benevolent while masking violence through ostensibly objective legal and scientific discourses. In practice, these clauses function as structural loopholes through which fundamental rights become conditional privileges – formally transforming universal duties of protection into discretionary powers exercised by professionals and institutions. Rights withdrawn precisely when protection is most needed exemplifies omission by commission operating at the legislative level.

Gurbai (2020) demonstrates how this approach has been endorsed by various treaty bodies. For example, he shows how the committees overseeing the ICESCR, and to some extent those overseeing CEDAW, have applied what might be termed a 'pragmatic definition' of discrimination. This definition legitimises differential treatment, including involuntary detention and forced treatment, whenever such interventions are deemed to pursue a legitimate aim and are considered reasonable by those in positions of authority. This exemplifies how commission by omission operates through international legal frameworks – granting authorities discretionary power to render fundamental protections conditional upon their own judgements. The UN CRPD Committee has, Gurbai (2020) notes, increasingly rejected this justification-based reasoning. Through General Comment No. 6 (UN CRPD Committee, 2018) and evolving case law concerning coercive psychiatry, the Committee is developing a position that disability-based deprivations of liberty and involuntary treatment are inherently discriminatory. They cannot be justified by appeals to public interest, protection, or therapeutic intent (Gurbai, 2020). This work by the UN CRPD Committee is vital. We hope that it will be ongoing.

Vague implementation obligations: The phrases 'progressive realisation' and 'to the maximum of available resources' when used in legislation or legal discourse are particularly problematic. They systematically transform immediate duties into indefinitely deferred obligations, representing omission by commission at the policy level. They allow states to justify failures to protect disabled people and guarantee their rights in terms of resource constraints. O'Sullivan and McNamara (2021) show how progressive realisation has been invoked to justify austerity measures, with governments like the UK enacting cuts that disproportionately harm disabled people. Thus, economic crisis serves as a shield against accountability.

Young (2019) argues that progressive realisation has normalised the idea of delay, resulting in rights-holders waiting indefinitely for entitlements that are legally recognised but deferred. Such waiting is not merely inconvenient – it can be tantamount to a denial of rights and allow the implementation or continuation of policies, programmes, or practices that are harmful to disabled people. For us, this mechanism perfectly exemplifies what Nixon (2011) terms 'slow violence' – harm that accumulates gradually, often invisible due to its incremental nature, yet no less destructive.

In a recent analysis, Clough (2025) has critiqued how legal frameworks – particularly around mental capacity and the CRPD – operate through static, fixed, and linear conceptions of time that legitimise delay, deferral, and stagnation in the realisation of rights. As she explains, '(o)ne of the reasons perhaps for such "glacial progress" in this context is the stagnant, fixed and static assumptions that often pervade the legal frameworks that the CRPD touches upon' (p 2). She argues that the CRPD has the potential to disrupt these problematic temporalities by jarring us 'out of existing temporal frames' (p 6) and creating an 'untimely orientation for future legal responses' (p 3). Her use of the concept of the 'untimely' is thought-provoking. This perspective directly supports our arguments about slow violence, progressive realisation as structural omission, and the legal legitimation of inaction through concepts like 'reasonable time'.

Medicalisation of disability: International and domestic legal frameworks continue to perpetuate violence against disabled people, particularly those with learning disabilities, psychosocial impairments, or neurodivergent identities, by legitimising coercive and exclusionary practices through the language of medical necessity and/or protection. This represents a sophisticated form of commission by omission – using medical authority to render fundamental rights conditional upon diagnostic categories and professional judgements about capacity. Returning again to the work of Clough (2017, 2022), she critiques the binary distinction between capacity and incapacity as a legal fiction that sustains control over disabled people's lives through subjectivation, infantilisation, and discretionary power. The CRPD, particularly General Comment No. 1 on Article 12, challenges this logic by affirming the right to legal capacity regardless of disability (UN CRPD Committee, 2014). Yet, most legal systems persist in using psychiatric diagnoses as grounds for substituted decision-making, involuntary treatment, and confinement – violence by commission reframed as therapy, assistance, or safeguarding (Minkowitz, 2007; FRA, 2012; Arstein-Kerslake and Flynn, 2016). In many jurisdictions, including across the EU, legal standards continue to allow detention for the protection of the person or others (FRA, 2012; Perlin, 2012), despite growing evidence that such thresholds are vague, inconsistently applied, and deeply traumatising for those subjected to them.

This laundering of violence through clinical language is not accidental. As Yergeau (2018) contends, diagnostic classification operates as a form of rhetorical violence, capturing neurodivergent lives in deficit narratives that strip away agency and intelligibility. Milton (2012) similarly explains how autistic-neurotypical communication breakdowns become pathologised as autistic deficits, legitimising coercive intervention and exclusion. Within mental health systems, LeFrançois et al (2013) and Burstow (2015) have shown that the very structures of psychiatry operate as systems of epistemic and embodied violence: institutionalisation, forced medication, and surveillance are enacted under the banner of care. These practices exemplify how ableism functions as a *dispositif* – an assemblage of legal, medical, and bureaucratic instruments that naturalise control while concealing harm (Foucault, 1980; Deleuze, 1992).

Drawing upon our book's typology, such mechanisms embody violence by commission (forced treatment), by commission by omission (denial of legal capacity by professionals with the authority to make such judgements), and via omission by commission (introduction of legal 'safeguards' that justify rights withdrawal). In this way, the law not only permits violence, it actively constitutes it through its selective recognition of personhood, capacity, and need. Beyond these concrete manifestations, our typology also acknowledges the foundational violence in the instituting moments of the *dispositif* – the dispersed processes through which it establishes itself as the dominant framework of intelligibility. The very act of transforming lived experience into diagnostic categories represents an epistemic violence that precedes and enables the more visible forms we have catalogued.

Lack of disaggregated data for purposes of monitoring: The absence of disability-specific data that would facilitate rights monitoring further obscures patterns of violence and limits the effective operation of legal frameworks. Lee et al (2022, p 2) highlight that 'very few countries report good quality, comparable, and consistent data' on disability. This data gap persists despite increased global interest and recognition of the importance of disaggregated data for policy and monitoring. The UN Department of Economic and Social Affairs (2024) recently acknowledged the absence of sound disaggregated data about the experiences of disabled people – it highlighted, for example, how limited data masks the greater risk among disabled women of experiencing intimate partner violence and raised concerns that disabled women remain invisible within policies, prevention, and response strategies.

A simple truth emerges: what remains uncounted remains invisible to legal bodies, legislators and policy makers. This erasure, we contend, constitutes a form of violence through omission at an institutional level – the systematic failure to fulfil duties of monitoring and protection that cannot be discharged without adequate data.

Normalisation of segregation: Despite international recognition of the right to community inclusion, separate systems in education, housing, and employment remain legitimised in many countries. This constitutes a form of spatial violence that we must acknowledge. Segregation is reframed as 'specialised provision' – a euphemism that masks its exclusionary nature. This represents omission by commission at the policy level – formal decisions to withdraw or withhold integration obligations while maintaining the fiction of adequate alternative provision. Rosenthal (2021) offers a compelling analysis of how conflicting interpretations of the CRC and CRPD perpetuate this problem. While the UN CRPD Committee (2017, para. 16[c]) has stated that '(l)arge or small group homes are especially dangerous for children, for whom there is no substitute for the need to grow up with a family. "Family-like" institutions are still institutions and are no substitute for care by a family,' the CRC continues to allow for placement in institutions as a form of necessary 'alternative care'. Article 20 of the CRC (1989) does not specify what 'alternative care' is acceptable/non-acceptable. Why does this matter? Because this contradiction enables what Rosenthal terms the 'medical/tragedy model' of disability to persist in international frameworks. As he observes, '(a)llowing the placement of the child in an institution, even as a "last resort", is a classic medical/tragedy model limitation on the child's rights based on actual or perceived deficits' (Rosenthal, 2021, p 111).

These competing standards – or more precisely, different 'interpretations' by UN committees – create barriers to recognising segregation (in this case in the form of institutionalisation) as violence.

Insufficient recognition of hate crimes: Lord et al (2024) observe that disability hate speech and crimes have until recently received very little attention from international institutions. The UN system has been particularly negligent in this regard. While there is now some traction in relation to addressing these issues, there is still much work to be done to ensure international human rights institutions account properly for disabled people within their work on hate speech and crimes. We consider it particularly troubling that the very frameworks designed to track violence have, to date, rendered the specific targeting of disabled people largely invisible. This invisibility allows such violence to continue unchallenged, representing a form of violence by omission – the failure of monitoring systems to fulfil their fundamental duties of recognition and response.

These mechanisms reveal how international legal frameworks, despite their stated commitments to protecting disabled people, often contain structural features that enable violence to continue unrecognised and unaddressed. The gap between formal legal protection and lived reality is stark. It reflects not simply implementation failures but conceptual limitations in how violence itself is understood within these frameworks. These limitations emerge through the systematic manipulation of duty relationships – transforming fundamental obligations into conditional privileges, deferring immediate duties through temporal sleight-of-hand, and formally withdrawing protections through policy decisions disguised as neutral administrations. As we have argued throughout this chapter, addressing these limitations requires a fundamental reconceptualisation of violence against disabled people.

Our typology offers a more comprehensive framework for identifying and addressing violence against disabled people, capturing forms of harm that often escape recognition within existing legal approaches. In the next section, we examine how the UN CRPD Committee's Concluding Observations provide empirical validation for our typology, demonstrating its relevance for understanding and addressing real-world patterns of violence against disabled people.

Empirical recognition: evidence from the UN CRPD Committee

While international legal frameworks provide normative standards for addressing violence against disabled people, examining how these standards are applied in practice reveals a chasm between promise and reality. The UN CRPD Committee – tasked with monitoring the implementation of this convention – provides a particularly rich source of empirical evidence through its Concluding Observations on State Party reports. These observations offer a window into disabled people's lived reality worldwide and the persistent, systematic violence they face – violence that is neither accidental nor isolated, but structural and pervasive.

To provide a contemporary picture, we have systematically analysed the Concluding Observations issued by the Committee between 2023 and 2025, covering more than 30 countries across both majority and minority world contexts. This approach has allowed us to identify patterns of violence that transcend national, economic, and cultural boundaries, demonstrating the universal nature of the problems we identify. The remarkable consistency of these patterns across diverse contexts speaks to the operation of a global system of ableism, rather than mere isolated occurrences of mistreatment or neglect. The universality of these patterns across different legal, cultural, and economic systems suggests that our typology captures systematic features of how ableism operates, rather than random policy failures. Table 2.2 captures our analysis, providing examples from Concluding Observations and encompassing countries from the minority and majority worlds.

Table 2.2: Types of violence recognised in UN CRPD Committee Concluding Observations with country examples

	Definition	Country examples from CRPD observations	Explanation (how it meets criteria)
Violence by commission	When someone does something directly harmful to a disabled person – includes hate crimes, all interpersonal violence, plus acts enabled by laws, institutions, or policies, such as the use of restraints, forced treatment, and sterilisation.	Argentina: Forced sterilisation of and abortions for women and girls with disabilities (CRPD/C/ARG/CO/2–3, para. 35).	Explicit act violating bodily autonomy.
		Germany: Use of restraints and seclusion in psychiatric facilities (CRPD/C/DEU/CO/2–3, para. 33).	Explicit institutional practices causing direct physical and psychological harm.
		Togo: Children subjected to inhumane treatment (CRPD/C/TGO/CO/1, para. 13).	Direct interpersonal violence.
Violence by omission	When people or institutions fail to act, leading to serious harm, such as not providing healthcare, not intervening in abuse, or not including disabled people in disaster plans.	Germany: No inclusive COVID-19 planning (CRPD/C/DEU/CO/2–3, para. 23).	Systematic neglect causing disabled people to face increased risk.
		Mauritania: No accessible evacuation protocols (CRPD/C/MRT/CO/1, para. 19).	Systematic neglect causing disabled people to face increased risk.
		Mongolia: Insufficient access to healthcare, assistive technologies, and devices (CRPD/C/MNG/CO/2–3, paras 23, 41, 47b).	Systematic neglect depriving disabled individuals of essential support.

Table 2.2: Types of violence recognised in UN CRPD Committee Concluding Observations with country examples (continued)

	Definition	Country examples from CRPD observations	Explanation (how it meets criteria)
Commission by omission	When someone with power and duty to protect or support a disabled person deliberately chooses not to act, enabled by discretion in laws or guidelines, thus causing harm or exclusion.	Germany (CRPD/C/DEU/CO/2–3, paras 21-22) and Israel (CRPD/C/ISR/CO/1, para. 21): Triage discretion during COVID-19.	Discretionary power legally enabling deprioritisation of disabled people for essential healthcare.
		Georgia: Family discretion to refuse life-saving care (CRPD/C/GEO/CO/1, para. 21).	Discretionary power legally enabling denial of life-saving care.
Omission by commission	When a law or policy actively removes, withdraws, or denies rights or protections from disabled people, explicitly withholding previously available or reasonably expected supports or rights.	Canada: Expansion of MAID eligibility removing previous protections (CRPD/C/CAN/CO/2–3, para. 19).	Explicit legal decision withdrawing critical protections safeguarding disabled people's right to life.
		Malawi: Expiry of National Action Plan on Albinism (CRPD/C/MWI/CO/1–2, para. 21b).	Deliberate policy decision removing previous legal protections and exposing people to discrimination and violence.
		Sweden: Legal restrictions explicitly removed personal assistance services from approximately 1,500 disabled individuals (2015–2022) and entirely excluded persons over 66 years from applying for such support (CRPD/C/SWE/CO/2–3, para. 41a).	Explicit policy action systematically withdrawing previously available essential support services, exposing disabled people to heightened risk of harmful institutionalisation and isolation.

The Committee do not explicitly use our typology; they speak in the language of rights violations rather than violence. Yet their observations provide compelling empirical validation for the categories we have identified. Reading between the lines of diplomatic language reveals a catalogue of violence against disabled people that precisely aligns with our four-part typology. What follows is not merely illustrative but evidential, empirical proof that our theoretical framework captures real-world patterns of harm.

These UN CRPD Committee observations represent real lives at risk of harm, damaged or destroyed, confirming that our typology captures real-world patterns experienced by disabled people across diverse contexts.

Four patterns emerge from this analysis:

1. **Violence by commission** is most consistently recognised, particularly when involving direct physical harm or explicit discrimination. Yet even here, the UN CRPD Committee often uses terms like 'mistreatment' or 'rights violations' rather than naming these practices explicitly as violence – a linguistic softening that, we suggest, fails to confront the embodied harm that wrecks lives.
2. **Violence by omission** receives less systematic attention, although the Committee increasingly highlights failures of inclusion. The causal link between these omissions and resulting harm often remains implicit rather than explicit.
3. **Commission by omission** is identified primarily in healthcare contexts, particularly around pandemic triage decisions. The Committee recognises the harmful effects of discretionary power but rarely frames such discretion itself as a form of violence – missing how professional authority systematically renders fundamental duties conditional upon ableist judgements about whose lives merit protection.
4. **Omission by commission** is addressed through concerns about regression in support services or legal protections. The Committee clearly recognises the harm caused by the active withdrawal of protections or support, but again without systematically conceptualising this as violence.

These patterns reveal a troubling reluctance to name violence against disabled people as violence, even within the most progressive international monitoring mechanisms. The Committee's consistent use of diplomatic euphemisms – 'mistreatment,' 'rights violations,' 'concerns' – reflects and reinforces the broader invisibility of ableist violence. When even expert bodies tasked with protecting disabled people's rights avoid confronting the violent nature of these practices, it demonstrates how deeply embedded these patterns of linguistic sanitisation have become. This systematic avoidance of the term 'violence' is not merely semantic but *political* – it obscures the severity of harm, diffuses responsibility, and maintains the fiction that these are administrative or technical failures rather than systematic attacks on disabled people's bodily integrity, autonomy, and survival.

This linguistic evasion, combined with the broader empirical findings from the UN CRPD Committee observations, raises fundamental questions about why these patterns persist so consistently across different legal, cultural, and economic contexts. The universality of these violations – their appearance across radically different legal systems, cultural contexts, and economic arrangements – suggests that legal frameworks alone cannot address violence against disabled people. Instead, we need to understand the deeper mechanisms that systematically produce, legitimise, and sustain these patterns of harm.

Understanding violence against disabled people

Disability Studies foundations

While our typology provides a framework for identifying and categorising different forms of violence against disabled people, it does not itself explain why and how these forms of violence occur and persist. The patterns we have identified demand a deeper explanation. To address this explanatory gap, we turn to theoretical frameworks that can illuminate the underlying mechanisms and drivers of violence. Before presenting our own theoretical approach, we briefly examine relevant contributions from Disability Studies and broader sociological traditions.

Within Disability Studies, violence has increasingly emerged as a central and critical concern, with scholarship illuminating its multiple dimensions: physical, psychological, epistemic, ontological, and institutional. Empirical analyses have demonstrated how disabled people are disproportionately subjected to harm within care homes, institutions, family settings, workplaces, and public spaces (Hughes et al, 2012). Hollomotz's (2012) work described a 'continuum' of violence, underscoring how seemingly benign everyday neglect or infantilisation easily escalates into explicitly harmful behaviours and profound psychological damage. There is now a substantial body of work on disability hate crime (see, for example, Sherry, 2010; Quarmby, 2011; Burch, 2021; and Burch and Wilkin [eds], 2024) that critically examines the lived experiences of disabled victims, along with the systemic failures of law, policy, and public discourse to recognise, address, or prevent such violence. Significant scholarship on carceral logics (for example, Ben-Moshe, 2020; Steele, 2020) has revealed how institutionalisation itself constitutes a form of structural violence – revealing how facilities ostensibly designed for 'care' function as sites of control, containment, and systematic harm. Violence permeates these spaces – it manifests through practices of restraint, isolation, and forced treatment that strip away dignity and autonomy. Steele's (2014, 2020) concept of 'lawful violence' powerfully underscores how ostensibly protective or therapeutic interventions are inherently violent through their denial of agency, autonomy, and consent.

In building our theoretical approach, we stand on the shoulders of these Disability Studies scholars who have provided crucial insights into specific manifestations of violence. Yet we believe that a comprehensive framework is still necessary to connect these varied forms of harm within broader networks of power/knowledge relations and material arrangements – an integration that our *dispositif* approach seeks to accomplish.

Theoretical development

In developing our theoretical framework, we integrate perspectives from several key sociological and philosophical traditions, each providing distinctive insights into how violence operates in relation to disabled people.

Walby's (2013; Walby et al, 2017) insistence that violence must produce measurable, embodied harm provides an essential empirical anchor for our analysis. While we depart from her requirement for physical contact, we maintain her focus on concrete, measurable effects rather than expanding violence into purely abstract domains.

Complementing this perspective, Žižek's (2008) distinction between subjective violence (visible, personal acts of harm) and objective violence (systemic harms arising invisibly from political and economic structures) offers valuable analytical tools. This distinction helps us recognise how violence against disabled people often remains unacknowledged precisely because it operates through taken-for-granted structures rather than spectacular events.

The temporal dimension of violence finds expression in Nixon's (2011) concept of slow violence, revealing how structural harms, neglect, and deprivation accumulate gradually, their devastating impacts obscured by their very quotidian nature. This concept proves particularly relevant for understanding how disabled people are subject to everyday violence – insidious in form and of accumulative toxicity. Unfortunately, when it comes to this 'slow' form of violence, the cause, ableism, is all too often obscured by the passage of time, along with the harmful consequences for disabled people's health and wellbeing. Like everyday racism or sexism, everyday ableism is not always recognised as violence. It proceeds under the radar. In addition to its accumulative toxicity, everyday ableism is, we argue, what makes 'faster' (escalation of) violence inflicted upon disabled people more possible and likely. This is where we incorporate Christian and Dowler's (2019) feminist relational approach to fast/slow violence as a single complex. Their work demonstrates how taken-for-granted violences become closely entangled with more explosive acts, supporting our conceptualisation of ableism as a *dispositif* of violence with both incremental and immediate manifestations.

For understanding the production of expendable populations, we turn to the work of Bauman on modernity and exclusion. In *Wasted Lives* (2004), Bauman examines how modernity produces certain populations as 'human waste' – individuals deemed excessive, redundant, or disposable. Disabled people, particularly those with significant support needs, frequently experience this categorisation – their lives positioned as burdensome within systems that prioritise productivity and standardisation.

The relationship between power, institutional practices, and the body is, of course, thoroughly explored within Foucault's work – and his work is our main source of inspiration. His analyses of disciplinary power and biopolitics (Foucault, 1991, 1998) offer powerful conceptual tools for examining institutionalised violence against disabled people. Institutions, such as schools, hospitals, and social care systems actively regulate and classify disabled lives, exerting pervasive forms of violence through institutional logics of exclusion, discipline, and normalisation directed at bodies deemed 'abnormal' or 'dependent'.

Developing Foucault's work further, Butler (2004, 2009) foregrounds normative frameworks that determine whose lives matter and whose do not. Her concepts of *precarity* and *grievability* demonstrate how normative hierarchies themselves function violently, through exclusion, dehumanisation, or neglect. Disabled people, rendered precarious precisely by ableist norms defining independence, productivity, and worth, experience this normative violence systematically and relentlessly when their lives are positioned as less grievable.

Finally, to ground our conceptualisation in concrete practices, we turn to David Sudnow's (1967) work on the social organisation of death and his analysis of how certain lives are deemed less valuable in medical decision-making. This concept of social death – where certain lives are devalued (made dead) before biological death occurs – connects powerfully with Bauman's analysis of 'wasted populations', and Butler's concept of differential 'grievability' helping us to understand how violence against disabled people is often normalised through professional judgements about quality of life or 'worth', for example, in terms of productivity.

Integration and application: theorising the violence complex

By integrating these theoretical perspectives, we can develop a framework that allows us to explore how our four types of violence function as part of an interconnected system. Rather than mapping theories to types in a one-to-one fashion, we adopt a bricolage approach, working with these perspectives to reveal the complex operations of violence against disabled people. This approach recognises that certain theoretical lenses are particularly relevant for specific types of violence while acknowledging their broader applicability.

Violence by commission encompasses both individual acts of interpersonal violence and institutionally sanctioned forms of harm. At the individual level, hate crimes against disabled people represent the most visible manifestations of this type, recognisable through Žižek's concept of subjective violence – direct harm with identifiable perpetrators. Yet importantly, these individual acts exist within a broader context of institutional responses that can function as a form of secondary violence. The failure of police to adequately investigate hate crimes against disabled people represents an institutional sanctioning of violence through what might be termed 'permissive neglect'.

Beyond individual hate crimes, violence by commission also operates through institutionally authorised forms of intervention. From a Foucauldian perspective, these apparently legitimate forms of violence – restraint, forced treatment, and sterilisation – operate through institutional practices that classify certain bodies as appropriate sites for control. Steele's (2014) concept of 'lawful' or 'legal' violence illuminates how these acts gain legitimacy through their authorisation within legal and medical frameworks.

Violence by omission operates not only through Nixon's concept of slow violence – harm that accumulates gradually over time – but can also produce immediate and catastrophic harm through acute neglect. The failure to provide accessible housing may lead to gradual social isolation and a decline in mental health, while the failure to implement appropriate supervision to keep a person safe can result in death within minutes. This dual temporality of omission – both slow and fast – is perfectly captured by Christian and Dowler's (2019) slow/fast violence concept.

Commission by omission manifests in both individual professional decisions and systematic institutional practices of discretionary deprioritisation. At the professional level, it operates through the social organisation of death (Sudnow, 1967). When a doctor places a DNAR order on a patient with learning disabilities without consultation, this represents a conscious choice to withhold potentially life-saving intervention based on judgements about 'quality' of life, or worse, the 'value' of life. Yet beyond individual clinical decisions, commission by omission also operates at systemic levels. During the COVID-19 pandemic, numerous countries implemented triage protocols that explicitly or implicitly deprioritised disabled people for life-saving care. This was achieved, not through exclusionary language but rather through seemingly neutral criteria that disproportionately disadvantaged those with pre-existing conditions. This reflects what Foucault (1998) terms 'biopower' – the regulation of populations through judgements about which lives are worth sustaining.

Omission by commission represents perhaps the most structurally embedded form of violence in our typology, operating through formal, explicit decisions to withdraw protection or support from disabled people.

This operates most visibly through what Bauman (1989) famously described as 'bureaucratic violence' – harm produced through administrative rationality rather than emotional hostility. Violence becomes morally invisible when carried out via a chain of bureaucratic steps. When legislation explicitly reduces disability benefits below subsistence levels or narrows eligibility criteria for personal assistance, these acts harm disabled people and constitute what Bauman terms the production of 'human waste' through bureaucratic processes.

The temporal dimensions of omission by commission are particularly significant. While the formal decision itself might occur at a specific moment, its effects unfold across multiple timeframes. The immediate consequence is often the abrupt termination of essential support, producing 'fast violence'. Yet these formal withdrawals also initiate longer trajectories of what Nixon terms 'slow violence' – a gradual deterioration in wellbeing, incremental erosion of independence, and cumulative damage to physical and mental health over months or years.

This theoretical integration reveals how violence against disabled people operates simultaneously across multiple dimensions – institutional, normative, temporal, and embodied. It demonstrates how apparently different forms of violence are in fact interconnected elements within broader systems that produce, sustain, and legitimise the devaluation of disabled lives.

Conclusion: from typology to *dispositif*

In this chapter, we have sought to define violence with clarity and precision because this is a political and analytical necessity. Violence is not merely interpersonal assault; it is often quiet and procedural, an action of a pen rather than a fist. Our typology captures distinct mechanisms of harm that operate through different temporalities and visibilities. Through concrete examples, we have illustrated how these different forms manifest in disabled people's lives – from hate crimes to institutional neglect, from discretionary denial of care to policy-driven withdrawal of support.

Our examination of international legal frameworks has revealed recognition of these forms of violence, but also mechanisms that systematically obscure violence through exceptions clauses, vague implementation obligations, ongoing medicalisation of disability, and capacity-contingent protections. Analysis of UN CRPD Committee observations provided empirical validation for our typology while highlighting the need for more systematic conceptualisation of violence against disabled people and articulation of harmful acts *as violence*.

Moving beyond typology to theory, we have developed an integrated analytical framework drawing upon multiple traditions to understand how violence operates simultaneously across institutional, normative, temporal, and embodied dimensions. This framework reveals how different forms of violence function as interconnected elements within broader systems that devalue disabled lives. Our analysis demonstrates how these different mechanisms of harm are not isolated phenomena but systematic manifestations of ableism – revealing the need for a comprehensive framework that can capture how various forms of violence operate as coordinated elements within a broader system of oppression. In the next chapter, we extend this analysis by conceptualising ableism itself as a *dispositif* of violence – a heterogeneous ensemble of discourses, institutions, practices, and material arrangements that systematically produces, normalises, and legitimises harm toward disabled people. This *dispositif* approach will allow us to explore how seemingly disparate phenomena are connected elements within a broader system that renders certain lives more vulnerable to harm than others.

Cutaway 1: Thinking together – on violence and resistance

Angharad: Miro, what do you hope readers will do with our typology of violence?

Miro: I hope they'll use it widely in practice. There's power in being able to categorise harm precisely – to say that something isn't just *unfair* but constitutes a specific form of *violence*.

Angharad: Yes, our four-part model gives people language to name what's happening. Distinguishing types of violence creates clarity. The point isn't simply categorisation but developing more effective responses.

Miro: Exactly. For example, when we identify commission by omission – deliberate decisions not to act despite having the power to do so – it allows us to target advocacy at those discretionary spaces where decisions are made.

Angharad: And when we recognise omission by commission – how formal policies actively withdraw protection or support – we can challenge those systematic decisions. This is where our theoretical framework becomes crucial.

Miro: Yes. I do remember struggling with the typology terminology though! Not the easiest of linguistic formulations.

Angharad: Indeed not! Yet despite the awkwardness, we needed terms that would capture these distinct mechanisms precisely. Moving beyond the typology itself, which theoretical concepts most resonated with you, Miro?

Miro: For me, Nixon's concept of slow violence was transformative. It articulated something I'd felt but hadn't found language for – how damage unfolds gradually over time for marginalised groups, often invisibly unless you're experiencing it. This is precisely what happens to disabled people – the steady accumulation of barriers, small indignities, and erosion of rights.

Angharad: That concept resonated strongly with me too. I found it particularly powerful when combined with Walby's empirical approach, which insists that violence must produce measurable harm.

Miro: Though we felt her emphasis on physical contact was limiting, and we needed to get past that, didn't we?

Angharad: Exactly. That's why conceptualising ableism as a *dispositif* of violence became so important – it captures how violence operates through interconnected discourses, institutions, and practices. It helps us see violence, not as isolated incidents, but as part of a coherent system that devalues disabled lives.

Miro: What gives me hope is that by understanding these mechanisms, we create possibilities for resistance.

Angharad: Yes. Because resistance is almost always possible. That's the hopeful message disabled people's movements have consistently demonstrated. Even within oppressive systems, there are opportunities to create change. And the more precisely we understand how violence operates, the more strategically we can resist it.

3

(Re)conceptualising ableism

The concept of ableism has gained increasing traction within Disability Studies over the past two decades. It provides a critical lens through which to examine societal norms, practices, and structures that privilege certain forms of embodiment while marginalising others. Scholars across various theoretical traditions have developed sophisticated analyses of ableism – Wolbring's (2008, 2012) concept of ableism as an 'umbrella-ism' encompassing many forms of oppression, Campbell's (2009) epistemological and ontological framework, Foucauldian approaches, Mad Studies and Critical Autism Studies perspectives. These diverse theoretical contributions have significantly advanced our understanding of how ableism operates across multiple registers, including discursive, material, institutional, temporal, and embodied.

Despite these important advances, a critical conceptual gap remains. While violence against disabled people is widely documented empirically, existing theoretical frameworks rarely position violence as constitutive of ableism itself – as central to its ontology. This chapter addresses this gap by reconceptualising ableism as a *dispositif* of violence – a heterogeneous ensemble of behaviours, discourses, institutions, architectural forms, regulatory decisions, laws, administrative measures, and scientific statements that systematically produces, normalises, and legitimises harm against disabled people.

We draw, of course, on Foucault's (1980) concept of the *dispositif*. We are, however, also drawn to Deleuze's (1992) creative interpretation of it. We argue that ableism operates through multiple, interconnected forms of violence – the very forms delineated in our typology in Chapter 2 – each functioning through different temporalities and modes of power. This typology examines how moral and legal duties to protect, support, or refrain from harming disabled people are violated, avoided, or systematically undermined. We believe that the *dispositif* framework has great analytical potential. It allows us to examine how ableism operates simultaneously through material arrangements, discursive practices, institutional logics, and subjective experiences. It enables us to trace how ableism produces both disability and ability as relational categories through mechanisms of normalisation, classification, and regulation. Most importantly, it allows us to comprehend connections between seemingly disparate forms of violence, revealing how they function as part of a coherent, although constantly evolving, system.

This chapter continues as follows: first, we survey current theoretical perspectives on ableism, acknowledging their significant contributions to our thinking, while identifying the specific limitation our framework seeks to address. We introduce the *dispositif* framework, demonstrating its analytical utility for understanding ableism. We then articulate our original conceptual contribution: ableism as a *dispositif* of violence, examining its context, components, and operations across multiple domains. We explore how this *dispositif* functions *within*, through internalised ableism and identify potential avenues for subversion and escape – points where resistance and transformation become possible. Finally, we explore the analytical and political implications of this framework, setting the stage for the case studies that follow in subsequent chapters.

By reconceptualising ableism in this way, we aim not only to enhance theoretical understanding but also to provide more effective tools for identifying, analysing, and challenging the multiple forms of violence that shape disabled people's lives. Our framework seeks to reveal connections that might otherwise remain obscured. It identifies points of intervention that are often overlooked and imagines possibilities for resistance that might otherwise be foreclosed.

Current theoretical perspectives on ableism

Campbell's (2009 and later) work represents perhaps the most comprehensive theorisation of ableism to date. Crucially, she clarifies that ableism and disablism are distinct. She articulates disablism in terms of overt discrimination towards disabled people, while defining ableism as 'a network of beliefs, processes and practices that produces a particular kind of self and body (the corporeal standard) that is projected as the perfect, species–typical and therefore essential and fully human' (Campbell, 2001, p 44).

This definition moves beyond individual attitudes or discriminatory actions to position ableism as a pervasive epistemological and ontological system. Campbell (2001, p 44) emphasises how ableism establishes normative ideals of ability and humanity, rendering disability a 'diminished state of being human'. We find her exploration of how ableist norms are internalised, sustained, and performed by disabled people themselves, including through what she terms the 'compulsion to emulate able-bodied standards' particularly helpful (Campbell, 2008, n.p.). This attention to internalisation adds crucial depth to understanding ableism's operation at the level of subjectivity.

Wolbring (2008) offers another influential perspective, positioning ableism as an 'umbrella-ism' that underlies other forms of discrimination. Wolbring's analysis is particularly insightful in highlighting how emerging technologies produce new forms of ableism. His concept of 'transhumanised' ableism captures how technological enhancements create new divides between those who can access enhanced abilities and those who cannot, drawing attention to ableism's historical contingency and adaptability.

Foucauldian approaches have profoundly shaped Disability Studies, offering theoretical tools that implicitly or explicitly theorise ableism without always naming it as such. We have been much influenced by work in this vein. These approaches have been proliferating, and we can only hope to give a flavour here. We value the work of Davis (1995), who traced the historical construction of 'normalcy' as a regulatory ideal, and Titchkosky (2003), who analysed how disability policy constitutes disability as a governable condition through narratives that reinforce normative ideals of citizenship. The work of Tremain (2017) and contributors to her edited volume *Foucault and the Government of Disability* (2005, 2015) has been inspiring, beginning with her (2005) introduction to this landmark text, where she conceptualises disability as an effect of biopower and governmental practices rather than a pre-existing reality. Campbell's (2015) contribution to the second edition of Tremain's collection explicitly discusses an 'ableist apparatus' – a diffuse set of practices that manage disabled people through binary classifications and normative judgements. All these ideas inform our thinking.

Further, Borg's work (2015, 2018, 2022) extends Foucauldian analysis to explore critique as a desubjugating practice at the limits of power. He examines how narrative expectations around disability enact epistemic and psychosocial violence while revealing possibilities for counter-conduct within ableist regimes. In his work 'Conducting Critique' (2015), Borg argues against reductive readings of Foucault that treat subjects as passively constituted by power, reminding the reader that Foucault (2007, p 47) himself said, 'Critique is the movement by which the subject gives himself the right to question truth on its effects of power and question power on its discourses of truth'. Elsewhere, Beckett and Campbell (2015) have been similarly influenced by Foucault's theorising on power and resistance in their analysis of the resistance practices of the disabled people's movement in the UK.

We find Foucauldian theorisation of resistance to be particularly useful, helping to explain how disabled people engage in forms of counter-conduct even within highly controlled spaces like welfare systems, education, or care institutions, thereby resisting the subjectivities (compliant, exceptional, tragic) that ableism attempts to produce. Collectively, these Foucauldian approaches illuminate how ableism operates through mechanisms of classification, normalisation, and subjectification and how resistance is possible. What they rarely do, however, is connect these mechanisms explicitly to violence.

Recently, contributions from Mad Studies have further enriched our understanding of ableism. Mad Studies research has provided vital insights into the entanglement of ableism with sanism – the privileging of rationality and normative cognitive processes. Thorneycroft (2020) demonstrates how they function as mutually reinforcing matrices of oppression rather than parallel systems, jointly constructing boundaries of normativity that govern both bodies and minds. This analysis reveals how binaries of sanity/madness and ability/disability co-constitute each other, maintaining hierarchies of humanness through interlocking regulatory mechanisms. Johnk (2021) takes this analysis further, arguing that these matrices are fundamentally colonial in nature, operating through 'race-ability' (drawing on the work of Ben-Moshe; see Chapter 5 for further discussion) to manage populations deemed threatening to normative social orders. Mad Studies scholars have been particularly attentive to how ableism operates through epistemic injustice – the systematic devaluation of mad-identified people's knowledge and testimony. As Castrodale (2017) illustrates, this epistemic violence manifests not only in psychiatric contexts, but also in educational systems that pathologise divergent ways of learning, perceiving, and expressing. These perspectives expand our understanding of ableism beyond physical and sensory norms to encompass the regulation of affect, perception, and cognition.

Critical Autism Studies has emerged as another significant theoretical strand, and one we find particularly exciting (O'Dell et al, 2016; Woods et al, 2018). Researchers in this field have explored how autism is discursively produced within systems of normalisation and pathologisation. O'Dell et al (2016) have argued that autism should be understood not as a fixed biomedical reality but as a category constructed within particular epistemic and political contexts. This approach shifts our focus from individual deficits to the normative frameworks that determine what counts as legitimate communication, social relations, and ways of being in the world. Ebben (2019) offers a particularly compelling analysis of how autistic people are positioned within what she calls 'ableist economies of doubt' – systems where their authenticity, agency, and self-knowledge are persistently questioned by clinical and research authorities. This concept resonates strongly with our *dispositif* framework, revealing how ableism operates through regimes of visibility and utterance that determine whose experiences are recognised as valid. Importantly, Shapira and Granek (2019) further extend this analysis through their examination of 'psychiatric cisgenderism–ableism' in the autism–transgender nexus, demonstrating how multiple systems of normalisation intersect to regulate bodies and minds at the margins of binary categorisations.

While both Mad Studies and Critical Autism Studies have highlighted, powerfully, the discursive dimensions of ableism, they also wrestle with questions of embodiment and materiality that cannot be reduced to discourse alone. This tension between discursive construction and material reality represents a persistent challenge across Disability Studies – one that significantly shapes how we theorise ableism itself. Post-conventional approaches have sought to address perceived limitations in both discursive and materialist accounts within Disability Studies. Shakespeare's (2013) critical realist approach represents one attempt to bridge this divide, although we believe it risks re-essentialising impairment. We feel more affinity with Feely (2016) and Gauci (2020), who propose Deleuzian approaches to reconciling materiality with anti-essentialism. Feely's (2016) analysis of the experiences of people with learning disabilities through Deleuze and Guattari's concept of 'assemblage' offers a path beyond the impasse between constructionism and materialism, suggesting that disability emerges through contingent arrangements of bodies, technologies, discourses, and institutions, without requiring an essential foundation. Similarly, Gauci (2020) develops a posthuman Disability Studies that conceives disability not as an individual property but as emergent from multiple, shifting relations of power, affect, and materiality. While these approaches offer valuable alternatives to essentialism without abandoning materiality, we have chosen to work with Foucault's concept of the *dispositif* to achieve similar objectives, arguing that it better centres the strategic and historically contingent organisation of power/knowledge that gives rise to ableism as a governing logic. We are, however, adopting Deleuze's (1992) innovative interpretation of Foucault's concept (see next section).

More recently, rich bodies of work have emerged examining intersections of disability with other axes of oppression, and we carry insights from this work into our analysis. Decolonial perspectives have extended ableism's theorisation by examining its entanglement with colonial logics and practices (Hutcheon and Lashewicz, 2020). DisCrit scholars have demonstrated how racism and ableism function as 'interconnected and collusive' normalising processes (Annamma et al, 2016, p 14), revealing how racial difference is pathologised and disability is racialised through institutional practices. Queer Disability Studies has examined how ableism intersects with heteronormativity, with McRuer's (2006) 'crip theory', which maps connections between compulsory able-bodiedness and compulsory heterosexuality, being a foundational text. We find, however, more contemporary work in Queer Disability Studies particularly helpful – for example, Abbott et al's (2025) critical research into how LGBTQIA+ disabled people navigate self-directed support schemes in England. Their work reveals profound tensions between personalisation, identity, and care, exposing how ostensibly empowering care arrangements frequently compel disabled people to suppress core aspects of their identity to maintain essential support services. Their findings show that significant numbers of LGBTQIA+ disabled people conceal their sexual orientation or gender identity from personal assistants, experience discrimination, and find their needs routinely overlooked within support systems. This research highlights how seemingly progressive systems of 'choice and control' can paradoxically constrain authentic self-expression through the structural conditions they create, leaving marginalised individuals to negotiate impossible trade-offs between personal safety, authentic self-expression, and access to essential care.

Finally, we look to temporal dimensions of ableism, which have been elaborated by scholars exploring how disabled people navigate normative expectations of time and progress. We are indebted to St. Pierre's (2015) analysis of 'straight–masculine time', which reveals how communication norms enforce ableist temporalities, while Kafer's (2013) theorisation of 'crip time' reminds us that alternative temporalities that resist linear progress narratives are possible. These temporal analyses demonstrate how time can function as an oppressive force – structuring and disciplining – but it can also be subverted, reclaimed, and reconfigured through resistant practices.

These diverse theoretical perspectives collectively reveal ableism as a system operating across multiple registers. Collectively, they offer a rich source of knowledge and conceptual tools. Nevertheless, we identify several limitations across these approaches. First, while existing frameworks acknowledge ableism's systemic nature, they do not always theorise its specific mechanisms. Second, while violence against disabled people is widely documented, existing theories rarely articulate violence as a constitutive force of ableism. Third, despite valuable efforts to bridge discursive and material aspects of ableism, many approaches continue to emphasise the discursive. Fourth, the temporal dynamics of ableism as violence – how it evolves, adapts, and reconfigures – remain underexplored.

Our reconceptualisation of ableism as a *dispositif* of violence seeks to address these limitations.

The *dispositif* framework: analytical advantages

In *The Confession of the Flesh*, Foucault (1980, p 194) defines the *dispositif* as 'a thoroughly heterogeneous ensemble consisting of discourses, institutions, architectural forms, regulatory decisions, laws, administrative measures, scientific statements, philosophical, moral and philanthropic propositions – in short, the said as much as the unsaid. The dispositif itself is the system of relations that can be established between these elements'.

In this book, we deliberately reject reductive translations or interpretations of the *dispositif* that treat it as a static, mechanical apparatus; instead, we portray it as a relational network through which power/knowledge circulates. In contrast to Agamben's (2009) more ontological rendering of the apparatus as a structure of capture, we follow Foucault and Deleuze (1992) in understanding the *dispositif* as a relational, strategic formation. We envisage a network of interconnecting lines, rather than a machine – these lines demonstrating how power relations operate not (simply) through top-down repression but through productive, capillary networks. These relations are not fixed but strategically mobile, continually reconfiguring in response to resistance.

Three critical aspects of the *dispositif* make it particularly suited for theorising ableism:

First, the *dispositif* is characterised by **heterogeneity** – it brings together diverse elements across discursive and non-discursive domains. This heterogeneity is valuable for understanding how ableism operates simultaneously through medical classifications, architectural barriers, legal regulations, cultural representations, and embodied experiences – producing various forms of violence through their complex interrelationships.

Second, the *dispositif* is **strategic** – it emerges in response to a specific historical 'urgency' or need. As Foucault explains, the *dispositif* has 'a dominant strategic function' (1980, p 195), addressing perceived social problems or crises. In the context of ableism, this strategic function manifests in the management of bodies and minds deemed problematic or somehow excessive – deploying violence as a mechanism of control, containment, and correction. This connects directly to Bauman's (2004) analysis of modernity's impulse to classify and exclude those deemed 'excess' or 'waste'.

Third, the *dispositif* is **processual** – it evolves over time, through what Foucault (1980, p 195) terms 'functional overdetermination' and 'strategic elaboration'. Never static, it shifts in response to challenges and resistances. This processual nature helps explain ableism's historical evolution from explicit eugenic violence to more subtle forms of exclusion and control.

Deleuze (1992) offers a creative interpretation of Foucault's *dispositif* that we find particularly rich in its analytical potential. It is from Deleuze that the idea of the *dispositif* as composed of multiple, intertwined 'lines' that constantly shift, intersect and diverge emerges:

Lines of visibility determine what can be seen and how things become visible or invisible. These lines shape which disabled bodies are rendered hypervisible through medical diagnosis or institutional categorisation, and which remain invisible or erased. They help us understand how some forms of violence become spectacularly visible while others, particularly the slow, incremental forms with cumulative toxicity, remain hidden.

Lines of utterance govern what can be said, who can speak, and how language constructs reality. For disabled people, these lines manifest in medical terminology that pathologises difference, bureaucratic language that categorises and thereby determines needs, or cultural narratives positioning disability as a tragedy or inspiration. These lines determine which forms of violence can be named as such and which are linguistically reconfigured as care or protection.

Lines of force represent underlying power relations that shape interactions and privileges. Within disability contexts, these include power dynamics between medical professionals and patients, care providers and recipients, or policy makers and those affected by their decisions. These lines are crucial for understanding how violence against disabled people is systematically produced through relations that determine who has the authority to act upon whom.

Lines of subjectivation determine how individuals form identities within the *dispositif*. Disabled people's subjectivities are shaped by diagnoses, treatments, and cultural representations – although they may also develop resistant subjectivities that challenge ableist norms. These lines help explain both how violence becomes internalised and how it might be resisted.

Thus, the *dispositif* is simultaneously about capture and the potential for escape. It contains what Foucault understood as points of resistance and what Deleuze and Guattari (2004) conceptualised as 'lines of flight'. These represent emergent possibilities for counter-conduct, practices through which disabled subjects refuse to be governed in this way, by this assemblage. These ruptures remind us that, while the *dispositif* may be pervasive, it is not impenetrable, immutable or inescapable; it always contains the possibility of its own subversion. The tension between containment and escape is precisely what makes the *dispositif* a dynamic rather than static concept, and what creates openings for transformative action.

The *dispositif* framework offers significant analytical advantages for understanding ableism: it captures complexity and interconnection, integrates discursive and material dimensions, emphasises historical contingency, acknowledges productive power, and creates space for resistance. By understanding ableism as a *dispositif* of violence, we can more precisely map its operations, trace its historical development, and identify possibilities for disruption and transformation.

Defining ableism as a *dispositif* of violence

We thus define ableism as a *dispositif* of violence that produces, normalises, and legitimises harm against disabled people through interconnected discourses, institutions, practices, and material arrangements. This *dispositif* of violence establishes and enforces normative standards of ability and humanity, positioning disability as a deviation requiring management, correction, or elimination. Violence – in the multiple forms elaborated on in Chapter 2 – is not incidental to this process but constitutive of it.

To fully understand ableism as a *dispositif* of violence, we must situate it within its broader historical–economic context while recognising its specific operational logics. Capitalism – not merely an economic system but a totalising social formation – provides the fundamental terrain upon which this *dispositif* emerged and continues to mutate. Very few places on Earth remain untouched by capitalism's influence. This is not to suggest that ableism is absent from non-capitalist or pre-capitalist societies. Rather, we argue that the dominant version of ableism today is inflected by capitalism, and capitalism has intensified, reorganised, and globalised ableism. As Puar (2017) argues, capitalism does not merely disable; it actively *debilitates* – producing conditions of slow, attritional violence that wear down bodies deemed unproductive. This idea, in dialogue with Rob Nixon's (2011) notion of *slow violence*, allows us to read debility and ableism as central mechanisms of capitalist control. These are not merely by-products of exclusion but instruments of governance, sustained through economic, medical, and social infrastructures. Industrial capitalism, as Oliver (1990) and Gleeson (1999) demonstrate, created the very category of disability. It established norms of productivity, efficiency, and standardisation that rendered certain bodies 'problematic'.

The capitalist mode of production demands bodies that can be disciplined, regulated, and made productive according to market imperatives. This creates conditions where non-conforming bodies become subject to classification, intervention, and management. Within this context, neoliberalism operates as a specific governmental rationality. It shapes how the *dispositif* of violence functions today. Neoliberal principles – individual responsibility, market-based solutions, privatisation of care, entrepreneurial selfhood, and cost-benefit rationalities – become components within ableism as a *dispositif* of violence. These manifest in resource allocation and support system structures. They determine how disabled bodies are assessed for economic utility and how disabled people come to understand their own worth. Goodley (2014) shows how neoliberal demands for self-sufficiency generate specific forms of psychic distress for disabled people. Simultaneously, they justify the withdrawal of collective support through the austerity measures that Ryan (2019) has so powerfully documented.

This relationship is not simply contextual but strategic. Mitchell and Snyder (2015) observe that neoliberal capitalism has shifted from overtly excluding disabled people to selectively incorporating certain disabled bodies (those that can most closely approximate norms of productivity and independence) – 'ablenationalism' – while intensifying exclusion for others. This adaptation demonstrates the *dispositif's* flexibility. Even as certain forms of inclusion emerge, the fundamental violence against those deemed insufficiently productive continues through reconfigured mechanisms.

Ableism as a *dispositif* of violence operates through several interconnected mechanisms within this context:

1. **Classification and differentiation**: This *dispositif* of violence produces impairment as a distinct category through medical, legal, educational, and

administrative classifications. These classifications determine who receives diagnoses, services, accommodations, or benefits, establishing boundaries between the 'normal' and the 'pathological'. Such classifications often function through acts of commission – active interventions that mark, separate, and segregate – as well as acts of omission, through the failure to recognise or accommodate differences that fall outside established diagnostic frameworks. DisCrit scholars have demonstrated how these classification systems are simultaneously racialised, producing what Annamma (2018) calls 'the pedagogy of pathologisation' that disproportionately targets disabled children of colour. This mechanism connects directly to what Bauman (2004) identifies as modernity's compulsion to classify, order, and separate 'human waste' – populations deemed excessive or disruptive to social order.

2. **Normalisation and correction**: This *dispositif* of violence establishes normative standards of ability, function, and behaviour, directing resources toward correcting or minimising perceived deviations. Rehabilitation, special education, play therapies, behaviour modification, and assistive technologies often aim to ensure that the disabled child or adult approximates non-disabled norms rather than valuing diverse ways of being. These normalising processes frequently deploy acts of commission (forced interventions) and commission by omission (deliberate withholding of support that does not serve normalising aims). As Clare (2015) and Kafer (2013) document, these normalising imperatives are often interwoven with heteronormative expectations, positioning non-normative sexuality and disability as twin targets for correction.
3. **Spatial and temporal organisation**: Ableism as a *dispositif* of violence arranges bodies in space and time, determining who can access which environments at what speeds, and the pace at which bodies must engage. Inaccessible buildings, segregated settings, productivity expectations, and waiting periods for services all shape where and how disabled people can exist. St. Pierre's (2015) analysis of 'straight–masculine time' reveals how expected communication rhythms exclude dysfluent speakers from participation, while Hamraie (2017) demonstrates how architectural norms literally build ableism into physical environments. This spatial–temporal organisation operates through acts of omission (failure to create accessible environments and interactions), commission (enforced segregation) and omission by commission (systematic policies that delay access to services).
4. **Knowledge production and expertise**: This *dispositif* of violence generates and privileges certain forms of knowledge about dis/ability while marginalising others. Medical, psychological, and educational expertise typically outweighs disabled people's experiential knowledge. This maintains professional authority over disabled people's lives. This

epistemic dimension employs acts of commission (imposing expert classifications) and commission by omission (deliberate exclusion of disabled people's perspectives from decision-making processes). Further, Hutcheon and Lashewicz (2020) have demonstrated how these knowledge hierarchies often reproduce colonial logics that devalue Indigenous understandings of mind–body difference.

5. **Resource allocation and distribution**: Ableism as a *dispositif* of violence determines how resources are allocated based on perceived worth, capacity, and potential. Cost–benefit analyses, quality-adjusted life years, employability assessments, and eligibility criteria reflect and reinforce judgements about which lives are valued. Resource allocation often involves acts of commission by omission (deliberate decisions by those with discretionary authority not to provide certain supports) and omission by commission (formal, blanket policies that withdraw resources from disabled people). Ryan's (2019) powerful analysis documents how austerity policies in England systematically withdraw support from disabled people, producing material harm through deliberate policy choices. This connects directly to what Butler (2004, 2009) identifies as the differential allocation of precarity – the systematic production of vulnerability in certain populations through policy decisions, resource withdrawals, and normative frameworks that determine which lives are worth sustaining.
6. **Identity formation and subjectivation**: This *dispositif* of violence shapes how disabled people understand themselves and are understood by others. Diagnostic categories, cultural representations, professional interactions, and social expectations all influence subjectivation (identity formation) and often encourage the internalisation of ableist norms. This dimension operates through more subtle forms of violence – the slow erosion of self-worth, the pressure to conform, and the constant requirement to justify one's existence. This process of subjectivation interacts with other systems of power and subjectification. As Schalk (2018) demonstrates, the construction of disabled bodyminds is always already racialised and gendered, producing distinct experiences at various intersections.

Internalised ableism: the *dispositif* operating within

We aim to further our discussion on the previous point (6) mentioned above. A particularly significant mechanism through which ableism as a *dispositif* of violence operates is internalised ableism – the process through which disabled people incorporate and reproduce ableist norms within their own sense of self (the process of subjectivation). Examining internalised ableism through Deleuze's reading of Foucault's *dispositif* reveals how external structures of power become internal psychological processes with material (embodied) consequences.

Through ***lines of visibility***, ableism as a *dispositif* of violence establishes what aspects of impairment are noticed, scrutinised, and marked as problematic – both by society and, crucially, by disabled people themselves. These lines determine which bodily or cognitive differences become hypervisible objects of concern and which remain unacknowledged. When disabled people internalise these regimes of visibility, they begin to view their own bodies and minds through the ableist gaze, constantly monitoring those aspects of their impairments deemed most visible or problematic by normative standards. Reeve (2012) strikingly illustrates this. She quotes 'Lucy', a disabled woman and respondent in her research, who describes selecting a red wedding dress: 'Because I didn't want to walk down the aisle again, all in my perfect white dress (…) realising that I wasn't perfect anymore (…) I didn't feel perfect anymore' (Reeve 2012, p 85). For 'Lucy', her imperfection is hypervisible. This represents the internalisation of ableist lines of visibility, where disabled people come to see themselves primarily through dimensions of difference marked as significant by others.

The ***lines of utterance*** within ableism as a *dispositif* of violence determine what can be said about impairment and by whom. Medical terminology, rehabilitation discourse, inspirational narratives, and tragic framing all constitute, so it would seem, legitimate ways of speaking about disability. Expressions of anger, pride, or claims to justice are often delegitimised as signs of a 'bitter and twisted disabled person' or 'uppity crip'. When these lines are internalised, disabled people can come to adopt these sanctioned languages to describe themselves – speaking of their bodies as 'broken', accepting medical labels uncritically, apologising for needs, or framing their own existence through tragedy or inspiration. The internalisation of these discursive rules produces a form of violence whereby disabled people's self-expression becomes constrained by ableist frameworks that limit how they can articulate their own experiences, even to themselves.

The ***lines of force*** within ableism as a *dispositif* of violence represent power relations that structure interactions between disabled and non-disabled people. These power dynamics – professional authority over patients, bureaucratic control over resources, architectural power to determine access – become internalised as psychological mechanisms. Disabled people can come to accept unequal power relations as natural, questioning their own judgement when it conflicts with professional opinions, accepting restricted access as inevitable, or taking responsibility for 'failure' to overcome barriers (Mason, 1990). This internalisation of ableist power relations represents a particularly insidious form of violence, where external coercion becomes unnecessary because disabled people have incorporated the very lines of force that maintain their marginalisation.

Perhaps most significantly, the ***lines of subjectivation*** within ableism as a *dispositif* of violence determine how disabled people understand themselves and form identities. These lines shape the kinds of subjects disabled people can become – often limited to roles as patients, clients, burdens, or inspirations. When internalised, these lines constrain how disabled people imagine themselves and their possibilities. As Reeve (2012, p 85) observes, internalised oppression directly restricts 'choices about who they can be, such as a potential parent, lover, worker, or student'. This internalisation produces what she calls a 'false consciousness' where disabled people accept these limitations as natural consequences of impairment rather than social constructions. The violence here lies in the foreclosure of potential identities and ways of being, as disabled people come to believe that certain roles, relationships, or achievements are simply not for 'people like them'. As Foucault (1982, p 789) stated, violence 'closes the door on all possibilities'.

Crucially, what makes internalised ableism such a powerful operation of ableism as a *dispositif* of violence is how these four lines work together, reinforcing each other through continuous cycles of self-policing, self-silencing, self-subordination, and self-limitation. This produces forms of violence that align with our typology from Chapter 2: active commission through self-criticism and the forceful suppression of needs or expressions; and omission through the neglect of one's own wellbeing and acceptance of exclusion as 'natural'.

This relational dynamic positions disabled people as unwitting enactors of violence against their own psychosocial wellbeing, while non-disabled people and ableist social structures function as enablers that create and sustain the conditions in which internalised ableism flourishes. As disability activist Micheline Mason (1990, n.p.) once wrote:

> Internalised oppression is not the cause of our mistreatment; it is the result of our mistreatment. It would not exist without the real external oppression that forms the social climate in which we exist. Once oppression has been internalised, little force is needed to keep us submissive. We harbour inside ourselves the pain and the memories, the fears and the confusions, the negative self-images and the low expectations, turning them into weapons with which to re-injure ourselves, every day of our lives.

Mason's formulation precisely captures how internalised ableism emerges directly from external structures of oppression, yet once internalised, it becomes a self-perpetuating form of violence with measurable psychological and emotional consequences.

Understanding internalised ableism through Deleuze's lines allows its operation as part of the broader *dispositif* of violence to be recognised. This deeper understanding helps explain why addressing internalised ableism requires more than individual psychological interventions; it demands transforming the *dispositif* itself through collective political action across multiple domains. In Chapter 4, we will explore how these internalised processes connect to interpersonal manifestations of ableism as a *dispositif* of violence, particularly through microaggressions that both reflect and reinforce the *lines of visibility, utterance, force*, and *subjectivation* that constitute ableism as a *dispositif* of violence.

The domains of ableism as a *dispositif* of violence

It is also important to understand how ableism as a *dispositif* of violence operates across multiple, interconnected domains, manifesting its mechanisms in particular contexts while maintaining its overarching strategic function:

Material and architectural: Physical environments, such as buildings, transportation systems, and urban spaces are designed around presumed non-disabled bodies and minds. Inaccessibility is not merely an oversight but a form of violence that excludes, marginalises, and endangers disabled people. The seemingly neutral design of stairs, standard doorways, or visual-only interfaces constitutes violence by omission – a failure to anticipate and accommodate diverse embodiments. When accessibility is deliberately removed or denied despite knowledge of its necessity, this becomes commission by omission or omission by commission (depending on the circumstances) – a more active form of exclusionary violence.

Institutional and administrative: Healthcare systems, social services, education, employment, and legal frameworks all embed ableist assumptions that produce harm through eligibility requirements, assessment protocols, support limitations, and procedural barriers. Institutional violence often operates through all four forms identified in our typology: commission (forced treatments), omission (service gaps), commission by omission (deliberate denial of accommodations by those with discretionary power), and omission by commission (policies that explicitly withdraw supports).

Discursive and representational: Language, media, cultural narratives, and academic disciplines (medical/health and psy-sciences) all too often construct disability as deficit, tragedy, burden, or inspiration. These representations shape public perceptions, professional practices, and policy decisions in ways that justify or normalise violence against disabled people. When television portrays disabled characters as either pitiable victims or inspirational overcomers, when medical textbooks present disability primarily as pathology, and when policy documents frame disabled people as costly burdens, they cause *real* harm by giving 'legitimacy' to an assortment of acts of violence within our typology.

Normative and ethical: Philosophical frameworks, ethical principles, and moral judgements that prioritise autonomy, productivity, or particular cognitive capacities over other forms of value and relationship contribute to the devaluation of disabled lives. These normative assumptions underpin decisions about resource allocation, treatment, and care. Bioethical paradigms that privilege independence and cognitive rationality systematically devalue disabled lives. When bioethical frameworks presume that certain cognitive capacities are prerequisites for personhood, when economic models value lives based solely on productive output, when moral reasoning excludes *inter*dependence as a core human value – these create the conditions for violence through commission by omission, where certain lives are deemed less worthy of protection or investment.

Intersectional and differential: Ableism as a *dispositif* of violence operates differentially across social locations, producing distinct forms of violence at the intersections of disability with race, gender, sexuality, class, and other axes of identity. For example, DisCrit scholars have demonstrated how racism and ableism function as 'interconnected and collusive' normalising processes (Annamma et al, 2016, p 14), collaboratively producing educational segregation, criminalisation, and pathologisation of students of colour. Erevelles and Minear (2010, p 128) trace how 'disabled people of color' are caught at the 'violent interstices of multiple differences'. Such intersectional analyses reveal how ableism as a *dispositif* of violence operates not in isolation but through and alongside other systems of power, producing different forms and intensities of violence across social locations.

Embodied and psycho-emotional: Ableism as a *dispositif* of violence shapes how disabled people experience their bodies and minds, often producing shame, anxiety, hypervigilance, and internalised ableism. These effects are not merely psychological but represent the embodied consequences of structural violence. Reeve (2012) and Thomas (2007) document how psycho-emotional disablism operates alongside structural barriers to produce internalised forms of violence, while Goodley (2014) theorises how neoliberal demands for self-sufficiency and productivity generate specific forms of psychological distress. The relentless pressure to appear 'normal', the need to minimise pain or fatigue to maintain employment, the strain of navigating inaccessible environments – all constitute violence that inscribes itself directly onto disabled bodies and minds, shaping subjective experiences and limiting possibilities for wellbeing.

Creating lines of flight: resistance practices

Our framework not only maps how ableism operates as a *dispositif* of violence, but also identifies points where it might be disrupted and its violence reduced. Following Walby's (2017) crucial insistence that violence causes real, measurable harm to bodies and minds, we emphasise that resistance practices are not abstract theoretical exercises but material interventions that tangibly improve disabled people's wellbeing and reduce their exposure to violence.

While governmentality offers valuable insights into how power operates through 'the conduct of conduct', we have chosen the *dispositif* framework specifically for its capacity to capture the heterogeneous elements through which ableism functions. Unlike governmentality's emphasis on the rationalities of governance, the *dispositif* concept – especially as interpreted by Deleuze – illuminates, in a helpful manner, how ableism operates simultaneously through material arrangements, discursive formations, and embodied experiences. Articulations of 'lines' of visibility, utterance, force, and subjectivation provide, we suggest, more precise analytical tools for examining how disabled bodies are rendered hypervisible in some contexts while invisible in others. Additionally, this framework's emphasis on strategic reconfiguration and potential for escape – 'lines of flight' – captures both how ableism adapts when challenged and how resistance emerges within its operations.

Following Deleuze and Guattari (2004), we understand 'lines of flight' as immanent movements within and against existing systems that produce measurable reductions in harm. For disabled people, these include:

Collective access practices: Disabled communities have developed concrete methods for creating accessible environments when institutional structures fail them. As Piepzna-Samarasinha (2018) documents, these practices directly counter the violence of omission by, for example, providing ramps, captioning, scent-free spaces, and quiet rooms that prevent the physical exclusion, pain, and sensory overload many disabled people otherwise experience. These interventions measurably reduce the harm caused by inaccessible environments, allowing disabled people to participate in social life without the physical and psychological damage of navigating hostile spaces.

Mutual aid and care collectives: Against the violence of omission by commission – the policy-driven withdrawal of support services – disabled communities have established networks of material support. Mingus (2017) and Piepzna-Samarasinha (2018) document how these systems provide essential personal care, medication access, food security, and housing support when formal systems fail. These networks directly counter neoliberal abandonment by ensuring disabled people receive necessary life-sustaining assistance, preventing the concrete harms of neglect: malnutrition, medication disruption, exposure to elements, and deterioration of chronic conditions. Research shows these networks measurably reduce hospitalisation rates, housing insecurity, and premature deaths among disabled community members.

Crip technoscience: When medical systems and their personnel withhold or deny adaptive technologies (commission by omission or omission by commission), disabled people create their own solutions. Hamraie and Fritsch (2019) document DIY ventilator modifications, insulin delivery hacks, and custom mobility devices that directly address life-threatening gaps in medical provision. These interventions concretely reduce pain, increase mobility, maintain vital functions, and prevent medical crises. During the COVID-19 pandemic, for example, such adaptations kept people alive when medical rationing threatened ventilator access (Reynolds et al, 2021). These practices demonstrate how disabled people actively create material conditions for survival when formal systems fail.

Political advocacy and litigation: Organised resistance to discriminatory policies directly counters the violence of omission by commission. Through class action lawsuits, legislative campaigns, and direct action, disability justice movements have secured concrete protections, including deinstitutionalisation orders that free people from abusive confinement (Ben-Moshe, 2020), anti-discrimination protections that preserve housing and employment (Heyer, 2015), and enhancements to social welfare systems (Prince, 2016). The struggle continues, but there is a history of collective action demonstrating the transformative potential of disabled people's resistance.

Disabled people and their allies should not, *of course,* be forced into these resistance practices. Nevertheless, we can learn much from their purposeful invention, their critique and their acts of defiance.

Conclusion

In this chapter, we have proposed a (re)conceptualisation of ableism as a *dispositif* of violence – a heterogeneous ensemble of discourses, institutions, practices, and material arrangements that produces, normalises, and legitimises harm against disabled people. This framework builds upon foundational work in 'studies in ableism' while offering, we suggest, additional analytical precision, historical depth, and political utility.

By drawing upon Foucault's *dispositif* concept and Deleuze's creative interpretation, we have mapped how ableism operates as a network, through multiple, interconnected lines and across diverse domains. We have traced how *lines of visibility, utterance, force,* and *subjectivation* shape disabled people's lives, possibilities, and relationships. We have connected these operations explicitly to the four forms of violence identified in Chapter 2. We have considered how these processes operate not only externally but from within, through internalised ableism – where disabled people themselves become unwitting perpetrators of violence against their own psychosocial wellbeing, with non-disabled people and ableist structures functioning as enablers of this harm.

Our approach is distinct in several ways. It bridges discursive and materialist approaches to disability by showing how linguistic formations, representational practices, built environments, professional cultures, institutional protocols, and economic systems work in concert to produce disablement. It emphasises that the ultimate consequence of these assemblages is not merely theoretical but manifests as real, embodied harm to disabled people's bodies and minds. It incorporates intersectional perspectives that examine how ableism operates through and alongside other systems of power, producing different forms and intensities of violence across social locations. It identifies not only mechanisms of oppression but also 'lines of flight' – possibilities for resistance and transformation that emerge from within and against ableism as a *dispositif* of violence.

The chapters that follow demonstrate this framework's analytical utility through detailed case studies across different domains: hate crime, domestic and sexual violence, and microaggressions (as part of a continuum) (Chapter 4); confinement (Chapter 5); assisted dying and terminalism (Chapter 6); and the failure of human services during the COVID-19 pandemic (Chapter 7). These case studies illustrate how ableism as a *dispositif* of violence operates in specific contexts, how its mechanisms adapt to different circumstances, and how resistance emerges within and against ableist systems.

The *dispositif* creates what we might term 'zones of differential resistance' – contexts where lines of flight are more or less constrained by material and institutional arrangements. Where resistance appears most limited – in spaces of physical confinement or at moments of life's termination – this constraint itself reveals the intensified operations of the *dispositif*. The relative scarcity of escape routes in certain domains signals not the absence of resistance but the concentration of ableism in its most totalising form.

Cutaway 2: Thinking together – on ableism as a *dispositif* of violence

Angharad: Miro, I'm interested in how this theoretical framework translates into practical understanding. How has conceptualising ableism as a *dispositif* of violence changed your perspective on your everyday experiences?

Miro: I don't think it *has* changed my perspective, so much as given me a conceptual architecture – a way to articulate what I already knew intuitively. When people speak to my partner or personal assistant instead of asking me directly, when buildings lack ramps, when policies cut essential services – I always recognised these happenings as being somehow *connected*.

Angharad: Yes, I think that's what makes the *dispositif* framework so powerful – it provides language to explain how these experiences are interconnected expressions of the same system. It reveals the connections between institutional practices, cultural attitudes, and individual behaviours that collectively devalue disabled lives.

Miro: Exactly. And it's helped me understand my own experiences in a new light.

Angharad: I've been wondering how understanding internalised ableism through this framework has impacted your self-perception. Has it, at all?

Miro: I think many people assume that because I'm confident and professionally successful, I haven't internalised ableism. But external markers of success don't reveal the internal landscape of doubt. For years, I hesitated to pursue certain opportunities because I had absorbed the idea that disabled people couldn't succeed in those spaces. That's the *dispositif* operating through self-limitation.

Angharad: I think that is precisely what makes the framework so valuable – it helps us to recognise these internalised boundaries as products of ableism rather than personal limitations. It also reveals how ableism reproduces itself even without explicit external enforcement, which is what makes it such a pervasive and effective system of oppression.

Miro: While you're deeply engaged with theory, I know your commitment to advocacy informs your work, Angharad. So how do you see this framework supporting resistance efforts?

Angharad: Deleuze's concept of 'lines of flight' is central here – it helps us to identify escape routes within seemingly totalising systems. When disabled people create mutual aid networks and adapt technologies when medical systems fail, these aren't just workarounds – they are challenges to the *dispositif* itself, creating alternative possibilities outside its logic and grip on our lives.

Miro: One practical concern I have is about translating this framework beyond academic circles. How do we ensure these concepts remain accessible?

Angharad: That's where concrete examples become crucial. Our case studies in subsequent chapters demonstrate how this framework 'works' to help us understand everything from microaggressions to medical rationing during the pandemic. When people see how it helps explain their lived experiences, I think, and hope, that the theoretical language will become less intimidating.

Miro: And perhaps that's the ultimate test of a theoretical framework – whether it helps people make sense of their experiences and identify points of intervention?

Angharad: Yes, precisely! The value isn't in the terminology but in what it lets us understand and do. The *dispositif* framework reveals connections between seemingly disparate experiences and, crucially, shows that even within the most oppressive systems, resistance is always possible. There are always cracks, always potential lines of flight. That's what gives me hope!

Miro: Me too.

4

From hate crimes to microaggressions

In the previous chapters, we have developed a typology and theoretical framework for understanding violence against disabled people and reconceptualising ableism. We have established that violence operates through multiple, interconnected forms deployed through a wide range of institutional arrangements, discursive practices, and material configurations. This chapter applies this theoretical framework to examine interpersonal manifestations of ableism as a *dispositif* of violence across a spectrum of intensity and visibility – from overt hate crimes to subtle microaggressions directed toward disabled people.

To briefly recap our typology from Chapter 2: acts of commission involve direct actions that cause harm; acts of omission involve harm caused through inaction or neglect; acts of commission by omission involve intentional withholding of action by an individual where discretionary power exists; and acts of omission by commission involve harm resulting from a formal blanket withdrawal of protection through policy or law. These four types of violence operate through various temporal dimensions and produce measurable, embodied harm to disabled people's bodies and minds.

Furthermore, as articulated in Chapter 3, ableism functions as a *dispositif* – a heterogeneous ensemble of discourses, institutions, practices, and material arrangements that produces, normalises, and legitimises harm against disabled people. This *dispositif* operates through '*lines of visibility*' (organising what can be seen); '*lines of utterance*' (governing what can be said); '*lines of force*' (representing power relations); and '*lines of subjectivation*' (shaping the forms of selfhood available to individuals).

While the forms of interpersonal violence discussed within this chapter may appear distinct in their visibility, intensity, and recognition, we argue that they reveal important connections as expressions of the same underlying *dispositif*. Drawing upon extensive literature across Disability Studies, criminology, and gender studies from diverse global contexts, we examine how violence against disabled people operates across a spectrum, from hate crimes to everyday microaggressions, revealing shared patterns of devaluation and institutional failure. These mechanisms reflect and reinforce the broader systemic operations of ableism as a *dispositif* of violence. Such violence represents clear violations of Article 16 of the CRPD, which obligates states to protect disabled people from all forms of exploitation, violence and abuse both inside and outside the home.

Expanding the boundaries: hate crimes and ableism as a *dispositif* of violence

Disability hate crimes remain significantly underreported and poorly addressed within criminal justice systems globally, despite extensive documentation of their prevalence and impact (Sin et al, 2009; Burch, 2021). The definitional boundaries of 'hate crime' present significant challenges, with legal frameworks often creating artificial distinctions between protected characteristics. As Burch (2021, p 211) argues, these limited conceptualisations fail to capture the 'diversity of experiences, feelings, and understandings' that constitute hate-based violence against disabled people.

Burch helps us to understand hate crime beyond conventional legal parameters. Applying affect theory, she demonstrates how 'hate circulates within normatively architectured spaces, becoming stuck upon those who are not deemed to fit properly and ultimately, marking them as out of place' (Burch, 2021, p 74). This affective framing echoes Foucault's concern with how power operates through spatial arrangements and normative judgements. Taylor et al (2012) explicitly frame policing failures in this area as institutional ableism, arguing they arise not from straightforward discrimination but from entrenched societal and institutional 'normalcy' that systematically devalues disabled lives. Their analysis draws explicit parallels between institutional failures in responding to disability hate crime and the institutional racism identified in the Macpherson Report (1999) following the murder of Stephen Lawrence in the UK.

The evidence of institutional failure is damning. Sin et al's (2012) evaluation of 14 English police services found widespread inconsistency in structures, policies, and staff understanding, with many services lacking dedicated hate crime officers or adequate training. In South Africa, Holness (2021) found procedural accommodations for disabled victims largely absent across criminal justice procedures. Meanwhile, in the Czech Republic, Walach and Petruželka (2024) found that police were insufficiently prepared to communicate with people with learning disabilities about their hate crime experiences. This troubling pattern across diverse international contexts reflects ableism embedded within institutional structures.

The 2007 UK case of Fiona Pilkington illustrates how different forms of violence operate simultaneously. Despite reporting over 30 separate incidents of targeted harassment to UK police, authorities failed to intervene adequately. This case exemplifies how institutional frameworks (omission by commission) create permissive conditions that enable individual officers to exercise discretionary authority not to act (commission by omission), even when aware of escalating harm. The systematic neglect ultimately led Pilkington, overwhelmed by despair, to take her own life and that of her disabled daughter, Francecca. Individual officers' decisions not to investigate were legitimised through formalised discretionary powers embedded within institutional policies that effectively rendered protection of disabled people conditional rather than mandatory.

Our understanding of hate crimes is further complicated by several interrelated concepts. Macdonald et al (2023) introduce 'hate relationships' rather than isolated incidents, revealing how disabled people often experience hate crimes within coercive, ongoing relationships with perpetrators who are frequently neighbours. This sustained, quotidian nature of harassment aligns with Nixon's (2011) concept of slow violence. A particularly insidious aspect is what Roulstone et al (2011) identify as the 'hate/vulnerability binary', where criminal justice systems frequently frame disabled victims as 'vulnerable' rather than targets of hostility, shifting focus from perpetrators' hate to victims' perceived deficiencies. This exemplifies how ableism operates through lines of utterance – governing what can be said, who can speak, and how language constructs reality.

The remarkable consistency of these institutional failures across diverse national contexts confirms they are not isolated incidents but manifestations of ableism as a *dispositif* of violence operating globally. This is not simply a case of individual prejudice but a systemic problem embedded in institutional practices worldwide.

Gender, disability, and violence

As is recognised in Article 16 of the CRPD, the intersection of gender and disability creates particularly heightened risks of violence, with international evidence confirming consistently higher rates of intimate partner violence, sexual assault, and domestic abuse among disabled women compared to non-disabled peers. Again, this pattern holds across diverse geographical contexts (see McCarthy et al's [2017] study in the United Kingdom, Riley et al's [2022] work in urban informal settlements in Mumbai, India, and Emerson and Llewellyn's [2023] extensive analysis across 29 low- and middle-income countries). García-Cuéllar et al's (2023) systematic review of international evidence found that disabled women face particularly stark disparities in levels of financial abuse, with 100% of studies showing an increased risk, and with physical violence, where 81.3% of studies showed an increased risk.

These patterns of victimisation reflect not simply the 'addition' of separate oppressions but the distinct ways that ableism and sexism interact to produce specific forms of violence – or, to use our conceptualisation, how ableism as a *dispositif* of violence interacts with other *dispositifs*, for example, that of sexism.

The mechanisms of this violence often directly target impairment and disability. Perpetrators exploit care dependencies, withhold medication or mobility aids, and use impairment or disability-specific verbal abuse (McCarthy et al, 2017; McCarthy, 2017; Mushimiyimana, 2018; Walter et al, 2024). As one participant in McCarthy's study reported: 'Because I had learning disabilities and needed support, he used to drive that in my face' (McCarthy et al, 2017, p 274). These tactics illustrate how intimate violence against disabled women operates through the same ableist logics that structure public hate crimes, with perpetrators exploiting socially constructed vulnerabilities while simultaneously reinforcing them.

McCarthy's (2017) work raises a particularly important question about the arbitrary boundaries between categories of violence against disabled women. She quotes one of her respondents in asking, 'What kind of abuse is him spitting in my food?' (McCarthy 2017, p 595) – highlighting how actions that might be classified as 'domestic violence' when experienced by non-disabled women are often virtually identical to what might be termed 'hate crime' or 'mate crime' when experienced by disabled people. These taxonomic distinctions, McCarthy (2017) argues, do not reflect meaningful differences in the violence itself but instead reflect the compartmentalised ways that professional systems respond to disabled people's experiences.

This insight directly supports our *dispositif* of violence understanding of ableism as operating across multiple domains through similar mechanisms. The woman with intellectual disabilities, whose partner controls her finances, humiliates her for her impairment and isolates her from support, experiences violence through the same ableist logics as the disabled person targeted by strangers in public. Both forms of violence reflect and reinforce normative judgements about disabled lives as less valuable; both exploit socially constructed dependencies; and both remain inadequately addressed by systems that frequently fail to recognise the specificity of ableist violence.

The barriers to help-seeking for disabled women are particularly revealing regarding how the *dispositif* operates. Walter et al (2024) identify multiple, compounding obstacles: inaccessible services, stigma in health and legal systems, and structural ableism and sexism that permeate support frameworks. These barriers constitute violence through omission – the failure to create accessible pathways to safety and justice – as well as commission by omission, when professionals consciously decide not to pursue interventions based on assumptions about disabled women's credibility or capacity. As Healy (2020, p 190) found from interviews with disabled victims, professionals often discouraged reporting: '(They told me – ed), with my memory problems, the court would throw it out'.

The field of domestic violence exemplifies how lines of visibility operate within the *dispositif* of violence. Disabled women's experiences of violence often remain invisible within mainstream domestic violence frameworks, while disability-specific forms of abuse may not be recognised as domestic violence at all. This invisibility reflects 'compulsory able-bodiedness' – the assumption that bodies are naturally able unless proven otherwise – combined with gendered assumptions about who constitutes a 'proper' victim of intimate partner violence. The result is that disabled women experiencing violence find themselves caught between systems, their specific experiences rendered unintelligible through dominant frameworks that fail to recognise the intersection of ableism and sexism.

Yet amidst these patterns of institutional failure, disabled women develop sophisticated strategies of resistance. As Mushimiyimana (2018, p 5) reports from Rwanda:

> Helping women with disabilities organise their own community groups has boosted their self-esteem. Being confident and conscious of their value as human beings is the starting point for becoming active members of the community and self-advocates, for reporting abuse, but also dreaming of a better future.

Such collective practices clearly represent 'lines of flight' – vectors of resistance that escape, redirect, or rupture established patterns within the *dispositif*.

Children, disability, and violence: institutional failures and cultural norms

Disabled children face disproportionate risks of abuse and neglect across all international contexts, with disabled girls especially vulnerable (Stalker and McArthur, 2012; Wissink et al, 2015; Helton et al, 2017) – a fact also recognised in Article 16 of the CRPD. This heightened risk appears consistently in Helton et al's (2017) US study, Wissink et al's (2018) analysis of institutional cases in the Netherlands and Makhoul Koury et al's (2025) international scoping review. Children with intellectual or learning disabilities face particularly pronounced risks of sexual abuse (Euser et al, 2016; Helton et al, 2017), often within supposedly protective settings. Wissink et al (2018) found that 73% of reported sexual abuse cases in Dutch state care involved children with intellectual/learning disabilities – a stark indictment of systems ostensibly designed to protect.

Flynn's (2020) analysis offers a powerful lens for understanding these patterns. She identifies that abuse and neglect of disabled children stem from a complex network of interlinked factors rather than any single cause. Abuse emerges from interactions between individual, familial, cultural, professional, and systemic elements – a web of relationships that resembles Foucault's conception of power as dispersed and relational. Within this web, cultural devaluation positions disabled children as deviant or less worthy of protection, while structural failures in professional responses create conditions where abuse remains unrecognised or unaddressed.

A particularly revealing aspect of Flynn's work is her examination of how proceduralism and managerialism operate within child protection systems. Standardised assessment frameworks frequently reduce disabled children to administrative categories, obscuring their complex lived realities and making it easier for signs of harm to be missed. These bureaucratic practices, while appearing neutral or efficient, mirror the reductive logics of medicalised approaches to disability. Flynn introduces a productive ambivalence around professional discretion in this context. She notes that while rigid procedures can constrain judgement and professional discretion is often preferred, such discretion is not always benign – it can reflect and reproduce ableist assumptions. As she puts it, discretion is 'usually conceptualised as "good" but is not always so' (Flynn, 2020, p 963).

The institutional response to the abuse of disabled children reveals further operations of the *dispositif*. Wissink et al (2015) identified significant barriers to disclosure and justice, including communication challenges, inadequate professional training, victims being viewed as less credible, and poor record-keeping. These failures constitute violence through omission – the failure to create accessible reporting mechanisms – as well as commission by omission, when professionals consciously decide not to pursue allegations based on assumptions about disabled children's reliability or worth.

The intersection of disability and care settings creates zones of exceptional risk. Euser et al (2016) found children with mild intellectual/learning disabilities in out-of-home care had nearly three times higher risk of sexual abuse than children in regular care. Residential settings proved especially dangerous. This pattern reveals how spatial technologies within the *dispositif* – the segregation of disabled children in specialised facilities – create conditions for violence, even as they are justified as protective or therapeutic.

These institutional arrangements cannot be understood through individualised frameworks alone. Flynn (2020, p 959) argues that 'culture is a contributing factor to not just the increased incidence of abuse (…) but differential treatment of disabled children in child protection systems'. Her analysis aligns perfectly with our *dispositif* framework, highlighting how networks of cultural assumptions, professional practices, and institutional arrangements collectively produce conditions where violence against disabled children is simultaneously more likely and less visible – a violent paradox at the heart of supposedly protective systems.

Institutional continuity across the violence spectrum

The continuity of the ableist *dispositif* becomes particularly evident when examining institutional responses across the spectrum of violence. The same police force that fails to recognise repeated harassment as disability hate crime – as in the Fiona Pilkington case – typically lacks protocols for addressing the 'lower-level' hostility disabled people face daily. Similarly, educational institutions that lack effective anti-bullying strategies for disabled students permit unchallenged microaggressions in classrooms and social spaces, with potentially devastating effects, including increased suicide rates among this student group (see Wei et al, 2016).

In both cases, the institutional failure is not simply one of omission but reflects the same underlying devaluation of disabled people's experiences within the *dispositif*. When a headteacher dismisses a disabled student's complaint about repeated 'jokes' as 'just teasing', they enact the same logic as the police officer who categorises targeted harassment as 'antisocial behaviour' rather than a hate crime. This institutional continuity reveals how the *dispositif* operates seamlessly across the spectrum of violence, with the authorities normalising both spectacular and subtle forms of harm through their responses – or lack thereof.

Microaggressions and the capillary level of the *dispositif*

At what Hall (2019) terms the 'low-level' end of this continuum of violence lie microaggressions – the subtle, often unconscious slights, snubs, and invalidations that permeate everyday interactions. It is to this end of the continuum that we now turn. Rather than representing a separate phenomenon from the hate crimes and interpersonal violence discussed previously, microaggressions constitute what Foucault might call the 'capillary level' of a *dispositif* of violence – the finest, most intimate spaces where power penetrates social life.

Microaggressions play a crucial role in the development and maintenance of internalised ableism – a phenomenon we explored in Chapter 3. When repeatedly exposed to subtle messages of devaluation, disabled people may begin to incorporate these external judgements into their self-perception. The relationship between external microaggressions and internalised ableism positions disabled people as unwitting perpetrators of violence against their own psychosocial wellbeing, while non-disabled people and ableist social structures function as enablers that create and sustain the conditions for this internalisation process. Microaggressions represent perhaps the most pervasive 'enabling conditions' – the subtle, everyday interactions through which ableist norms are communicated, reinforced, and ultimately turned inward as self-judgement.

When examined through our typology of violence, microaggressions facilitate internalised ableism through multiple mechanisms. Microaggressions as acts of commission (unwanted help, invasive questions) provide the raw material for internalised negative self-beliefs. Microaggressions as acts of omission (exclusion from conversations or failure to provide accessibility), communicate to disabled people that their participation is not essential or expected, leading to internalised beliefs about their own unworthiness. Perhaps most insidiously, microaggressions as acts of commission by omission – such as medical professionals deliberately dismissing pain reports – reinforce internalised ideas that disabled people's experiences are not to be trusted, even by themselves.

Through the lens of our *dispositif* framework from Chapter 3, we can observe that microaggressions operate primarily along lines of subjectivation, shaping how disabled people come to view themselves and their possibilities. The disabled person who has repeatedly experienced patronising 'you're *so* inspirational' comments for achieving ordinary activities may begin to internalise this as a pressure to do *more* – feeling obligated to exceed expectations just to be valued and accepted. When friends thoughtlessly organise gatherings in inaccessible venues, the excluded disabled person may begin to see themselves as 'the problem' – an inconvenience whose needs disrupt otherwise smooth social interactions. These processes reveal how microaggressions transform external ableism into internalised self-limitation and self-blame – a particularly insidious operation of ableism understood as a *dispositif* of violence.

Understanding and evidencing microaggressions as violence

The concept of microaggressions has evolved significantly since psychiatrist Chester Pierce first introduced the term in 1970 to describe subtle insults directed at Black Americans. Building on this foundation, Sue et al (2007, p 271) developed a comprehensive taxonomy, defining microaggressions as, 'brief and commonplace daily verbal, behavioral, or environmental indignities, whether intentional or unintentional, that communicate hostile, derogatory, or negative racial slights and insults toward people of color'.

Within disability contexts, Keller and Galgay (2010) were among the first to systematically apply this framework, identifying disability microaggressions that included denial of personal identity, denial of disability experience, and infantilisation. Their research demonstrated how disabled people routinely encounter interactions that minimise their experiences or assume incompetence. Kattari's (2020) subsequent *Ableist Microaggression Scale* provided empirical evidence correlating these experiences with psychological harm.

While these frameworks have advanced understanding of subtle discrimination, *on the whole,* they have limitations when viewed through our theoretical lens. Conventional approaches tend to frame microaggressions primarily (if not exclusively) as interpersonal phenomena rather than systemic issues. Moreover, by categorising microaggressions based on form, rather than function or impact, traditional taxonomies may obscure how seemingly different interactions produce similar harm through different mechanisms. Our reconceptualisation addresses these limitations by understanding microaggressions within our typology of violence and the broader *dispositif* of ableism, examining how everyday interactions are shaped by, reinforce, and sometimes disrupt broader configurations of power, knowledge, and materiality.

For us, Kattari's (2019, 2020) work represents a significant advancement in studying ableist microaggressions and remains our touchstone. Through mixed-methods research, she developed the *Ableist Microaggression Scale* to measure both the frequency and impact of microaggressions experienced by disabled people. This work provides crucial empirical evidence of their harmful effects, moving beyond theoretical claims to document tangible impacts on disabled people's wellbeing.

Kattari's approach integrated multiple theoretical frameworks, drawing on social dominance theory (Sidanius and Pratto, 1999), critical race theory, and stigmatisation theory (Goffman, 1968a) to understand how microaggressions reflect and reinforce broader social hierarchies. Through a carefully designed multi-phase research process, she developed the AMS-65, a 65-item scale that captures the breadth and complexity of ableist microaggressions across multiple domains, including exclusion from social or public life, invalidation of disability experience, stereotypical assumptions of helplessness, ableist language or jokes, assumptions of inferiority, intrusions on privacy, and ableist assumptions about sexuality and reproduction.

Perhaps most significantly for our analysis, Kattari's research provides compelling evidence that ableist microaggressions are not merely offensive or uncomfortable but constitute forms of violence that produce measurable harm. Her studies demonstrate strong statistical correlations between the frequency of ableist microaggressions and adverse mental health outcomes, including increased depression, heightened anxiety, difficulty with behavioural control, and reduced positive affect (Kattari, 2020). These relationships remain robust even when controlling for participants whose primary impairments are psychosocial, indicating that the harm of ableist microaggressions extends across impairment categories rather than simply reflecting pre-existing mental health conditions.

These findings do, of course, align with Walby et al's (2017) insistence that sociological analyses of violence must remain grounded in empirical evidence of embodied harm rather than abstract theorisation. By documenting the tangible, measurable impacts of microaggressions on disabled people's mental health and wellbeing, Kattari ensures that discussions of ableist microaggressions remain connected to their lived consequences rather than descending into theoretical abstraction. Moreover, her empirical approach reinforces the political urgency of addressing microaggressions – not as trivial slights or mere insensitivities but as forms of violence that systematically harm an already marginalised population.

Microaggressions through our typology and *dispositif* framework

In this section, we want to reconceptualise ableist microaggressions through our typology of violence and the *dispositif* framework. We offer a more comprehensive analysis that illuminates how everyday interactions both reflect and reinforce broader ableist structures. This approach, we suggest, extends and enriches existing frameworks rather than replacing them. It provides additional tools for understanding and challenging microaggressions as manifestations of ableism as a *dispositif* of violence.

Our typology of violence (see Chapter 2) facilitates the identification and articulation of ableist microaggressions as they operate through diverse mechanisms. Microaggressions, as acts of commission, include direct verbal or behavioural slights. These include the use of ableist language, overt verbal abuse, and uninvited or unwanted touching, such as forcibly assisting people with visual impairments or the inappropriate use of assistive devices, such as sitting on the armrests of wheelchairs or pushing people without their consent. They also include making derogatory jokes, expressing pity, or treating disabled people as objects of inspiration. Such microaggressions actively inflict harm even when taking seemingly benign forms like unwanted help or excessive praise.

Microaggressions, as acts of omission, involve failures to acknowledge, include, or accommodate disabled people due to inaccessible environments, lack of information in accessible formats, social gatherings organised without consideration of accessibility, or interpersonal omissions such as directing questions to non-disabled companions. These cause harm through what is *not done,* reflecting implicit assumptions about expected, or 'ideal', abilities, who belongs, and whose needs deserve consideration.

The more complex forms operate through systemic processes: commission by omission involves deliberate decisions not to act despite awareness of potential harm. For example, when a conference organiser consciously ignores accessibility concerns; when someone chooses to ignore fragrance-free requests ('It's just a little perfume!'); when someone deliberately withholds accommodations ('I prefer this meeting isn't hybrid, so you must attend in person'); or knowingly deprioritises disability as part of diversity initiatives in the workplace. The harm arises not from ignorance but from a calculation that the issue does not warrant attention. Finally, omission by commission involves systemic and systematic, blanket approaches. For example, bureaucratic requirements to repeatedly prove impairment, even for long-term conditions, to be able to access certain support, institutional priorities of efficiency or cost-cutting over accessibility ('Only some doors in this new building open automatically/have push button openings'), or professional training perpetuating ableist assumptions under the guise of expertise.

The last of these examples warrants particular attention here because of the critical role professionals and professional knowledge play within the *dispositif*. Medical training that teaches healthcare providers to view disability primarily as a deviation from normal functioning rather than as a valued form of human diversity, leading to interactions where professionals assume their patients will welcome lengthy, painful interventions in order to become 'more normal'. Psychology training that focuses on disabled children's 'play dysfunctions' and the role of play in their 'normalisation', leading to therapists developing 'playful' interventions that transform children's play into a *work* activity. Education programmes that frame neurodivergent learning styles as 'problems to manage', rather than different ways of processing information, resulting in teachers who unconsciously communicate lower expectations to neurodivergent students. Customer service training that categorises disabled customers as having 'special needs', encouraging staff to apply 'extra patience', setting up interactions where staff display exaggerated helpfulness or speak in infantilising tones. Architectural and design education that treats accessibility as a technical compliance issue rather than a fundamental design principle, producing professionals who view accessibility features as afterthoughts or compromises to aesthetic vision. Law enforcement training that characterises mental health crises as primarily a matter of public safety threat rather than a health emergency, leading to interactions where officers respond to distress with control tactics rather than support.

We know that not all professional training programmes perpetuate ableism in this way, but those that do create distinct 'lines of force' within the *dispositif* – institutionalised pathways through which professional authority over disabled people is simultaneously legitimised and naturalised. By connecting these seemingly disparate professional contexts, we can identify how microaggressions operate not as isolated, interpersonal failings but as systematic expressions of ableism as a *dispositif* of violence that positions disabled lives as less valuable, less complete, and less worthy of accommodation than their 'able-bodied', 'normal' counterparts.

By connecting microaggressions to broader forms of violence, this typology resists their trivialisation as mere insensitivities, underscoring their role in sustaining systematic oppression through mechanisms that extend beyond individual intention to institutional structures and practices. Beyond categorising microaggressions through our violence typology, we propose understanding them as operations within the broader *dispositif* of ableism. Returning to Deleuze's (1992) interpretation of Foucault's *dispositif* concept, we can understand microaggressions through the four interrelated 'lines' that we discussed in-depth in Chapter 3.

Lines of visibility determine what can be seen and how things become visible or invisible. Within the ableist *dispositif*, microaggressions contribute to patterns of hypervisibility and invisibility – rendering some impairments spectacles of difference while erasing or minimising others. Consider how certain impairments become objects of unwanted attention through intrusive questions or staring, while invisible impairments are all too often invalided or dismissed. Both patterns reflect how the ableist *dispositif* manages visibility, determining which bodies and experiences can be seen and acknowledged, and under what conditions.

Lines of utterance govern what can be said, who can speak, and how language constructs reality. Ableist microaggressions often govern discourse, subtly silencing disabled voices while privileging professional or non-disabled perspectives. When medical practitioners dismiss disabled people's accounts of their own experiences, when academic settings fail to include disability perspectives within curricula, or when social conversations minimise disability-related concerns, these microaggressions enforce specific rules about whose speech matters and what can legitimately be said about dis/ability. They are not merely offensive comments but practices that establish and maintain discursive boundaries within the *dispositif*.

Lines of force represent the power relations that structure interactions between different subjects. Microaggressions frequently manifest these power dynamics through professional authority over disabled patients, bureaucratic control over resource allocation, or social privilege to define what constitutes 'normal' behaviour or appearance. When employers assume incompetence, when healthcare providers make unilateral decisions about treatment, or when strangers offer unsolicited advice or assistance, these microaggressions reveal and reinforce power imbalances embedded in the *dispositif*. At this capillary level, microaggressions represent the everyday manipulation of basic duties (primarily moral but sometimes legal), eroding fundamental obligations not to harm, exclude, or invalidate others through seemingly minor but accumulative violations of interpersonal responsibility.

Lines of subjectivation determine how individuals understand themselves and others. Microaggressions influence identity formation by continuously communicating messages about worth, capability, and belonging. For disabled people, persistent exposure to invalidation, pity, or assumptions about limitation can foster internalised ableism – a sense that one's differences are indeed deficiencies. For non-disabled people, participating in microaggressions reinforces their subject position as 'normal', capable, invulnerable, and authoritative. In both cases, microaggressions operate as technologies of the self, shaping how individuals understand their place within social hierarchies.

From a *dispositif* perspective, the documented mental health impacts of microaggressions reflect how they operate as technologies of power – not merely offending but *disciplining* bodies and minds. When disabled people develop heightened vigilance, self-doubt, or social withdrawal in response to persistent microaggressions, these psychological adaptations serve to limit their participation and reinforce their marginalised status. The cumulative nature of these impacts aligns with Nixon's (2011) concept of slow violence – a toxicity that accumulates incrementally, becoming visible only through longitudinal examination.

As previously mentioned, Reeve's (2012) research on psycho-emotional disablism demonstrates how this internalisation process directly restricts who disabled people can be and become, as they incorporate external limitations into their self-concept. This restricted sense of possibility represents perhaps the most profound harm of microaggressions – they not only wound in the moment but also constrain people's future horizons.

This analysis reveals how microaggressions function as more than interpersonal failings; they are enactments of ableism as a *dispositif* of violence – mechanisms through which broader systems of power, knowledge, and materiality operate at the level of everyday interaction. They reflect not merely individual prejudice but institutional logics, professional norms, cultural representations, and spatial arrangements that collectively constitute ableism as a pervasive social phenomenon.

Crucially, understanding microaggressions as operations within the ableist *dispositif* allows us to recognise their relationship to other forms of violence against disabled people. Microaggressions connect to broader patterns of exclusion, discrimination, and harm – not as separate phenomena but as manifestations of the same underlying *dispositif* operating at different scales and through different mechanisms. The medical professional who dismisses a disabled patient's concerns because they can, the architect who designs inaccessible spaces because they overlooked the needs of disabled people, the policy maker who cuts disability benefits, and the stranger who abuses a disabled person on public transport are all enacting elements of the same *dispositif*, albeit through different types of violence.

Implications for practice and resistance

Reconceptualising interpersonal violence against disabled people through our typology of violence and the *dispositif* framework has significant implications for both practice and resistance. Our analysis reveals that addressing the spectrum of violence – from overt hate crimes to subtle microaggressions – requires interventions at multiple levels, targeting not only individual behaviours but also the broader structures that sustain and legitimise harm against disabled people. The institutional practices, cultural attitudes, and systemic arrangements that enable violence must be confronted alongside individual instances of harm.

Addressing hate crimes and institutional failures

For criminal justice professionals, our framework emphasises the need to recognise connections between seemingly 'low-level' incidents and more severe hate crimes. This understanding challenges police practices that categorise repeated harassment as merely 'antisocial behaviour' rather than recognising its hate-based motivation. Training programmes should focus not only on identifying individual incidents but also on recognising patterns of escalation and the continuum of violence that Hall (2019) describes.

The institutional failures documented across countries highlight the need for structural reforms in policing. We suggest that these should include:

- Specialised training on disability hate crime recognition that addresses the 'hate/vulnerability binary' (Roulstone et al, 2011), which frames disabled victims as inherently vulnerable, suggesting violence towards them is almost inevitable, rather than acknowledging them as targets of hostility.
- Clear protocols for responding to repeated incidents targeting disabled people.
- Accessible reporting mechanisms that accommodate diverse communication needs.
- Multi-agency coordination between police, healthcare providers, and disability organisations to ensure comprehensive responses.

As Taylor et al (2012) argue, failures to respond appropriately reflect systemic ableism embedded within institutional structures rather than simply individual prejudice. Reform efforts must therefore address the foundational assumptions that devalue disabled lives within criminal justice systems globally. These institutional failures represent violations of disabled people's rights under the CRPD, particularly Article 13 (access to justice), which requires states to ensure effective access to justice for disabled people on an equal basis with others. The persistence of hate crimes also reflects broader failures to implement Article 8 (awareness-raising), which obligates states to combat stereotypes and prejudices that fuel violence. Addressing hate crimes thus requires not only improved criminal justice responses but also systematic efforts to transform the cultural attitudes and institutional practices that enable such violence.

Gender-based violence and intersectional approaches

For those working to address violence against disabled women, our analysis highlights the need for intersectional approaches that recognise how ableism and sexism, along with multiple other forms of oppression, interact to produce specific forms of violence. Practical interventions should include:

- Training for domestic violence service providers on disability-specific forms of abuse, including exploitation of care dependencies and withholding of medication or mobility aids.
- Accessible refuge services and helplines for disabled women experiencing violence.
- Recognition of disability-specific forms of abuse within domestic violence assessment tools and interventions.
- Supporting community-based approaches like those documented by Mushimiyimana (2018) in Rwanda, where disabled women's self-organised groups have boosted their self-esteem and enabled them to become self-advocates.

These approaches recognise what Walter et al (2024) identify as the compounding barriers disabled women face – inaccessible services, stigma or lack of awareness within healthcare and legal systems, and isolation.

Child protection and institutional care

Our examination of violence against disabled children highlights the need for fundamental reforms in child protection and alternative care systems. The evidence is overwhelming and unequivocal: institutions are dangerous places for disabled children. They constitute sites of heightened risk where violence through all four forms in our typology frequently occurs. We must be absolutely clear: what is needed is not reform of institutional care, but rather complete deinstitutionalisation, which must be accompanied by proper investment in community-based living and family support.

Flynn's (2020) analysis of how ableist cultural norms, professional practices, and institutional frameworks contribute to disabled children's elevated risk of abuse calls for interventions that:

- Challenge the proceduralism and managerialism that reduces disabled children to administrative categories, obscuring their complex lived realities, while simultaneously maintaining close scrutiny of practices associated with professional 'discretion'.
- Develop disability-inclusive safeguarding practices that address the specific risks faced by disabled children, particularly those with learning disabilities.
- Move urgently toward complete deinstitutionalisation with significant investment in community-based alternatives, rather than merely attempting to reform residential settings.
- Create accessible disclosure and reporting mechanisms that recognise communication differences and ensure disabled children can report abuse.

These reforms must address the cultural factors contributing to the differential treatment of disabled children in child protection systems – challenging the deeply embedded assumptions and stereotypes that cloak neglect and normalise violence. Without such fundamental cultural change, procedural reforms alone will prove insufficient.

Addressing microaggressions and everyday hostility

At the 'capillary level' of the *dispositif*, addressing microaggressions requires interventions that recognise their role in sustaining broader patterns of violence. Drawing on Kattari's (2020) empirical research linking microaggressions to adverse mental health outcomes, these approaches should:

- Recognise microaggressions as forms of violence that produce measurable harm rather than dismissing them as mere insensitivities or over-sensitivities on the part of the victim.
- Develop educational programmes that help non-disabled people to recognise and challenge their own ableist assumptions and behaviours.
- Support disabled people in developing strategies to navigate and resist everyday hostility, including collective practices of solidarity and validation.
- Create institutional policies that address the systemic nature of microaggressions as part of our culture rather than treating them as individual behavioural issues.

For professionals working with disabled people, our framework emphasises the need to examine not only explicit attitudes but also institutional logics, procedural requirements, and environmental configurations that may produce microaggressions through systemic mechanisms. Entire professional systems may be organised in ways that systematically devalue or marginalise disabled people's experiences. This examination requires moving beyond individual competence toward institutional transformation.

Collective resistance across the violence spectrum

Our framework provides disabled people with both analytical tools and strategic insights for resistance. By understanding interpersonal violence as a manifestation of a broader pattern of ableism as a *dispositif* of violence, rather than as isolated incidents, disabled individuals can contextualise their experiences within broader systems of oppression, potentially reducing self-blame and isolation.

We agree with Burch (2021) – resistance can be seen in the very act of survival. Merely existing, persisting, and asserting one's presence in a world structured to exclude, can constitute a form of resistance. These everyday acts of persistence and self-assertion, sometimes barely perceptible yet profoundly significant, represent 'lines of flight' – vectors of resistance that escape, redirect, or rupture established patterns within the *dispositif*.

We suggest that survival is not enough; disabled people need to be able to *flourish*. Collective resistance strategies might therefore include:

- Disabled people's organisations challenging hate crime legislation and implementation, as we have seen in the work of the UK's *Disability Hate Crime Network*.
- Women-led initiatives, such as those documented by Mushimiyimana (2018) that create spaces for disabled women to support each other and advocate against violence.
- Self-advocacy groups for people with learning disabilities that challenge institutional care practices and demand rights-based approaches to support.
- Collective development of counter-narratives, including those that harness the evocative and provocative potential of arts practices, to challenge ableist assumptions about disabled lives as inherently less valuable or worthy of protection.

Such practices recognise a fundamental truth – individual interventions alone cannot address violence against disabled people. Momentary acts of recognition or awareness-raising, while valuable, remain insufficient. What is required is a sustained challenge to the broader *dispositif* that sustains and legitimises harm against disabled people across social systems.

Conclusion

By reconceptualising interpersonal violence against disabled people through our typology and *dispositif* framework, we have offered a comprehensive approach to understanding and addressing the full spectrum of harm experienced by disabled people – from overt hate crimes to subtle microaggressions. Our analysis reveals how these apparently distinct forms of violence operate through the same underlying mechanisms, reflecting and reinforcing a broader system that devalues disabled lives. The connections between different manifestations of violence are neither coincidental nor superficial; they are structurally embedded within the *dispositif*.

The implications for practice and resistance are profound, requiring interventions at multiple levels – individual, institutional, and systemic. By recognising the interconnections between different forms of violence, we can develop more effective strategies for challenging the *dispositif* that sustains and legitimises harm against disabled people. These strategies must centre disabled people's voices and experiences, recognising their agency and resilience in the face of systemic oppression.

This continuum of interpersonal violence, however, does not exist in isolation from broader institutional arrangements. As already touched upon in this chapter, microaggressions that police disabled bodies in public spaces, or that diminish the credibility of disabled speakers, find their most extreme expression in formal systems of segregation and control. In the next chapter, we shift our focus to the issue of confinement – the institutional practices that physically separate disabled people from mainstream society. As we will demonstrate, the same *dispositif* of violence that operates through interpersonal hate crimes and everyday microaggressions also functions through these more formal structures of containment and exclusion.

Cutaway 3: Thinking together – from hate crimes to microaggressions

Angharad: Miro, we've explored this spectrum from hate crimes to microaggressions theoretically, but I wonder if you'd share some of your own experiences with microaggressions and their impact on your wellbeing?

Miro: It's the cumulative effect that's most exhausting. When people speak to my PA instead of me, express surprise that I work, or tell me I'm 'inspiring' for doing the shopping – each instance seems minor, but together they create this constant background noise of being treated as 'Other'.

Angharad: That slow, accumulative impact is precisely what Nixon's concept of slow violence helps us understand, isn't it?

Miro: Absolutely. After particularly draining days – navigating an inaccessible venue, being told someone 'couldn't live like that', or hearing I'm 'so brave' – my body physically reacts. My shoulders tense, my breathing changes, sometimes I develop migraines. The psychological toll translates directly into physical symptoms, which validates Walby's point about violence producing measurable, embodied harm.

Angharad: I'd like to ask about your experience delivering training on disability hate crime. What key messages do you most want to communicate?

Miro: The most crucial thing is helping people understand that what they dismiss as 'antisocial behaviour' or 'bullying' often constitutes targeted, hate-motivated crime against disabled people. The same incidents police might categorise as 'low-level nuisance' can have devastating impacts when experienced repeatedly.

Angharad: The Pilkington case is particularly significant here, isn't it?

Miro: Yes, it exemplifies exactly what we're discussing. Fiona Pilkington and her disabled daughter Francecca experienced years of targeted harassment, and reported it over 30 times, but police consistently categorised it as 'antisocial behaviour'. The failures of recognition ultimately led to their deaths. When I share that case in training, it often creates a moment of realisation about how institutional failures to recognise disability hate can have fatal consequences.

Angharad: How have professionals typically received this training?

Miro: It varies enormously. Some have those 'lightbulb moments' where they suddenly recognise patterns they've missed. Others become defensive, insisting they 'treat everyone the same' without recognising that standardised responses often fail disabled people. The most resistant are usually those who've been working longest in their fields – they've internalised professional frameworks that fundamentally misrecognise ableist violence.

Angharad: That resistance confirms how deeply embedded ableism is within institutional practices – exactly what our *dispositif* framework would predict. I've delivered hate crime training to police forces from three European countries, and several officers claimed they didn't believe disability hate crime existed because people would feel 'so sorry for disabled people they wouldn't want to be cruel to them'. This complete misunderstanding of how ableism operates shows just how pervasive these misconceptions are.

Miro: That doesn't surprise me. It's the same infantilising attitude that sees us as objects of pity rather than targets of hostility.

Angharad: Exactly. And I've encountered similar denial in schools. Teachers earnestly insist, 'We don't have any bullying of disabled children here; all our children are very kind,' which is completely at odds with reality! They genuinely don't recognise what's happening as ableist bullying. They've normalised it as 'just kids being kids' or rationalised it as something the disabled child must have provoked.

Miro: And interestingly, when I train across different sectors – police, healthcare, education – I see the same patterns of minimisation and misrecognition, just expressed through different professional languages.

Angharad: That consistency across sectors supports our argument that these aren't isolated failings but manifestations of the same underlying *dispositif.* How do you think our approach might be useful for practitioners?

Miro: What's powerful about our approach is how it connects seemingly disparate phenomena. When training police officers, they often struggle to see connections between hate crimes, 'everyday' microaggressions and institutional practices. Our framework demonstrates that the officer who dismisses repeated harassment as 'just antisocial behaviour' is participating in the same *dispositif* as the doctor who speaks to a PA instead of the disabled patient or the teacher who organises a school trip to an inaccessible venue despite knowing of the access needs of a member of their class.

Angharad: So it creates a more comprehensive understanding of how ableist violence operates across different levels?

Miro: Yes, and importantly, it moves beyond individual blame. When we talk about institutional ableism, practitioners often become defensive. But our *dispositif* framework shows how they're operating within systems that shape what they can see, say, and do. It creates space for structural change rather than just individual awareness training, which rarely produces lasting transformation.

Angharad: That's a crucial insight about why awareness training alone is insufficient.

Miro: The framework also validates disabled people's experiences by showing how microaggressions, institutional neglect, and hate crimes are connected manifestations of the same underlying structure rather than isolated incidents.

Angharad: Theory and practice aren't separate worlds, are they? What gives me hope about our approach is that it offers both analytical precision and practical insight – a framework that helps understand ableist violence while simultaneously identifying points where intervention might be most effective. That's the ultimate test of theory, isn't it? Its ability to illuminate not simply what is, but also what might be otherwise?

Miro: Yes, indeed.

5

Confinement: institutions and disabled children/youth

> The phrase 'out of sight, out of mind' is no longer acceptable. I am going to talk to you about my life in institutions, foster homes, and care services. I am in your sight today. (Martin, 2019, p 1)

We open with these powerful words by Sir Robert Martin, the New Zealand disability activist, leading member of the global self-advocacy movement, and person with a learning disability who grew up in institutions and foster care. In 2016, Sir Robert was elected to the UN CRPD Committee. He served on this committee until 2024, when he sadly passed away. He is much missed by all who knew and admired him. We dedicate this chapter to his memory and begin each section with a quotation from his powerful testimony to the Royal Commission of Inquiry into Abuse in Care (1950–1999), New Zealand.

In this chapter, we explore how ableism operates as a *dispositif* of violence through formal systems of segregation and control. Confinement represents a curious paradox: simultaneously more visible as an institutional manifestation of violence, yet often rendered invisible because it is seldom acknowledged as violence at all. Instead, it is justified through ostensibly benevolent discourses of care and protection, obscuring its true nature behind a veneer of therapeutic or other 'necessity'.

The critique of the confinement of disabled people has long been central to both critical Disability Studies and survivor-led movements. Much of the academic literature – and certainly most of the legal, policy, and practice frameworks – has focused on adults, especially those confined in psychiatric hospitals, large congregate care settings, or carceral institutions. Goffman's (1968b) foundational concept of the 'total institution' and Wolfensberger's (1975) typology of devalued roles have shown that institutionalisation is not merely a question of place, but of power, surveillance, and social death (Calabria and Cullen, 2024). The problem extends beyond physical architecture and encompasses the social relations, power dynamics, and dehumanising processes that constitute institutional life.

Deinstitutionalisation policies, influenced by the Independent Living Movement and disability rights activism, have sought to dismantle large institutions in favour of community-based living. Despite this policy shift, more than 1.4 million disabled people in Europe were still living in residential care as of 2019 (Šiška and Beadle-Brown, 2023). Many live in settings for more than 30 people, with people with learning disabilities remaining especially vulnerable to lifelong institutionalisation (Šiška and Beadle-Brown, 2023). The trend towards the so-called 'home turn' – supporting people in their own homes – has not resolved these problems. Research shows that home or community settings may reproduce institutional features when support is inadequate, rights remain conditional, and personal autonomy is limited (Ben-Moshe, 2011).

Without parallel investment in accessible, rights-based services, the closure of psychiatric hospitals has, for example, often contributed to a form of reinstitutionalisation. This occurs via prisons, group homes, or prolonged hospitalisation under a different guise (Fulone et al, 2021; Calabria and Cullen, 2024). Many disabled people simply move from one form of segregation to another. The institutional logic remains intact despite changes in physical settings. Disabled children and youth are particularly vulnerable, often caught in these transitional logics – receiving the language of inclusion but the lived experience of confinement.

This chapter's focus on children and youth is intentional. While extensive research examines the institutionalisation of disabled adults, the specific experiences of disabled children and youth have received far less sustained academic attention. This oversight is problematic because childhood represents a period of distinct vulnerability. Disabled children – as a population with limited legal standing, political voice, and capacity to resist – experience ableism as violence in particularly acute ways. Their confinement illustrates not only individual instances of harm but also a broader system that deems certain lives less valuable, certain bodies as requiring containment, and certain futures as expendable. We frame confinement not simply as exclusion from space, but as denial of full personhood.

Critical insights from the psychiatric survivor movement and Mad Studies become particularly relevant here, as survivor-led work emphasises that coercion often begins young – through educational labels, diagnostic regimes, and early psychiatric interventions. Many children grow up in systems denying them the right to refuse treatment, to be heard, or to live outside institutions. This matters deeply for our focus on childhood, as early confinement shapes life trajectories and can determine whether someone becomes permanently institutionalised.

Our approach builds upon Bauman's (1997) conception of 'human waste', where institutionalisation serves as the paradigmatic example of what he terms 'anthropemic strategies'. These are the mechanisms through which modern societies 'vomit the strangers, banishing them from the limits of the orderly world' (Bauman, 1997, p 18). We extend this analysis to include Ben-Moshe's (2020) conceptualisation of carceral logics, which encompasses the rationalities justifying confinement in the name of care, safety, or protection.

Such logics operate through our typology of violence. Together, they create a system rendering disabled children simultaneously hypervisible as objects of intervention yet invisible as subjects with rights.

We intentionally include evidence from multiple countries to underscore the global nature of this problem. We will, nevertheless, return repeatedly to a particular UK case – that of Connor Sparrowhawk. Connor, affectionately known as 'Laughing Boy' by his family, was a young man with autism, epilepsy, and learning disabilities who loved buses, music, and recycling. He died on 4 July 2013, drowning in a bath at Slade House, a short-term assessment and treatment unit run by Southern Health NHS Foundation Trust. Despite his known epilepsy and previous seizures, the staff reduced their observations. An inquest jury found that his death was entirely preventable.

Connor's death matters deeply to us. His mother, Sara Ryan, is a highly respected member of the Disability Studies community in the UK, whose advocacy we admire. We approach his case not as detached observers but as engaged scholars who see politically committed research as central to the emancipatory tradition in Disability Studies. By weaving Connor's story throughout our analysis, we honour all those who have suffered under institutional regimes.

Connor's case reveals how ableism, as a *dispositif* of violence, operated through all four lines (as introduced in Chapter 3) simultaneously. *The lines of visibility* – which determine what can be seen and how things become visible or invisible – caused the institution to render Connor hypervisible as a 'risky' patient requiring management, while systematically ignoring his family's intimate knowledge of his epilepsy and care needs. *The lines of utterance* – which govern what can be said and who can speak – enabled the institution to privilege medical discourse over family expertise, as documented during the investigation into Connor's death (Verita, 2014). *The lines of force* – representing power relations that structure interactions – manifested through institutional authority that overrode family concerns about seizure risks in favour of standardised protocols that ultimately failed Connor. *The lines of subjectivation* – which determine how the *dispositif* categorises and constitutes individuals as particular types of subjects – functioned within the institutional setting to redefine Connor primarily through medical categories of deficiency and risk, rather than recognising him as the young person with interests, relationships, and unrealised possibilities that his family knew him to be.

Theorising confinement: beyond 'care' to carceral logics

> Just because I was born with a disability. I was being punished just for being who I was. (Martin, 2019, p 6)

To understand institutions for disabled children as sites of confinement rather than benevolent care, a conceptual shift is required. Despite decades of deinstitutionalisation efforts, the segregation of disabled children continues under various guises, justified through discourses of protection, treatment, or specialised care. While acknowledging that care relationships can be meaningful, we argue that institutional environments fundamentally transform these relationships through carceral logics and power dynamics. As Ben-Moshe (2020) argues, these justifications mask fundamentally carceral rationalities, determining who should be separated from society, surveilled, and subjected to control.

The lines of our *dispositif* framework materialise with particular clarity in institutional settings: *lines of visibility* determine which disabled bodies are seen as requiring containment; *lines of utterance* establish professional discourses that justify confinement as care; *lines of force* manifest in direct control over disabled children's bodies; and *lines of subjectivation* shape how disabled children understand themselves within these confining contexts.

Series' (2022) analysis of the 'institutional archipelago' extends Foucault's (1991) concept of the 'carceral archipelago' and is particularly helpful here. She reminds us that this archipelago includes traditional institutions alongside community-based services, special schools, assessment units, and supposedly therapeutic environments. What connects these spaces is not their physical architecture but the underlying disciplinary logic that positions disabled bodies and minds as objects requiring intervention.

Series (2022, p 8) observes that 'What begins as "safeguards" for individual liberty can become the cutting edge of new forms of power'. This paradox is evident in ostensibly protective legal frameworks – such as capacity assessments and best interests decisions – that can function, we argue, as mechanisms of violence by commission, enabling direct control over disabled people's lives while claiming benevolent intent. These frameworks do not simply fail to protect; they actively authorise confinement, treatment, and surveillance that would be recognised as violence if imposed on non-disabled people without such legal cover.

When applied to institutional settings for disabled children, our typology allows us to grasp how confinement operates through multiple forms of violence:

Commission: direct acts of restraint, seclusion, forced medication, or physical discipline that actively inflict bodily harm.

Omission: the failure to provide stimulation, education, proper care, or meaningful social interaction, negatively impacting upon children's development and wellbeing.

Commission by omission: application of professional discretion in ways that deny necessary accommodations, medical treatment, or education based on assumptions about disabled children's capacity or worth.

Omission by commission: systematic, blanket-approach policies or practices that withdraw protection or support, such as resource allocation models that prioritise institutional over community-based care or legal frameworks that facilitate confinement with minimal oversight.

These forms of violence are not aberrations within otherwise benevolent systems but constitutive elements of how ableism functions as a *dispositif* of violence in institutional contexts. They reflect and reinforce broader cultural, political, and economic logics that devalue disabled children's lives and justify their spatial, social, and legal segregation from normative society.

While we believe that children are particularly vulnerable, we in no way deny their capacity to resist. We recognise the complex personhood of disabled children in confinement. Disabled children cannot be reduced to passive victims, pathological bodies, or subjects of care. Rather, they inhabit multiple, sometimes contradictory subject positions: they resist, accommodate, and transform the institutional spaces they occupy; they form relationships, assert themselves, and maintain dignity, even within systems designed to deny those possibilities. The ways in which their agency is 'interpreted', however, may limit the potential of their resistance, such as when it is understood in terms of 'problem behaviour' or 'acting out' and then efforts are made to control their actions.

The production of confinement: classification, differentiation, and disposability

> We were not given our own clothes. We had to share a pool of clothes and grab what we could get. We never had our own underwear. They didn't let us just be a kid. We were colour-coded in groups and had [...] labels and categories. We all had the same bowl haircuts on the same day. We were not treated as individuals. (Martin, 2019, pp 6–7)

The path to institutionalisation begins long before a child enters a residential facility. It starts with processes of classification and differentiation that mark certain children as different, deficient, or dangerous – as requiring specialised interventions and separate spaces. These processes operate through what Foucault (1982, p 777) terms 'dividing practices', which simultaneously individualise subjects through close examination and categorise them into groups based on perceived similarities.

For disabled children, these dividing practices often take the form of diagnostic procedures, developmental assessments, and educational evaluations. While presented as objective and scientific, these classifications function as 'lines of utterance' within the broader operation of ableism as a *dispositif* of violence – they establish who can speak about disability, what can be said, and which knowledge counts as authoritative. The consistent prioritisation of professional knowledge over family expertise or children's own experiences represents a form of epistemic violence that creates the conditions for physical confinement.

From a UK context, Connor Sparrowhawk's case illustrates precisely this epistemic violence. Despite his mother's intimate knowledge of his epilepsy and support needs, her expertise was systematically devalued within the institutional setting. As documented in the subsequent investigation and inquest, 'families felt like they were treated as the enemy' (Verita, 2014, p 84) – a sentiment that reflects the broader tendency of professional systems to dismiss experiential knowledge in favour of clinical evaluation. This devaluation of family expertise directly contributed to the circumstances of Connor's death, as family warnings about his seizure risk were disregarded in favour of institutional assessment protocols.

The systematic over-representation of disabled children in out-of-home care demonstrates how they become channelled towards confinement. A comprehensive scoping review by Shannon et al (2023), examining seven countries – the US, UK, Netherlands, Canada, Spain, Israel, and India – found that children with intellectual and developmental disabilities (IDDs) are disproportionately placed in institutional settings rather than family-based care. Their review documented how in one study '1 in 6 parents of children with IDDs had considered placing their child in OOHC [out-of-home-care] (…) due to increased care needs, lack of resources to provide care, and pervasive impact on the entire family' (Shannon et al, 2023, p 16). This reflects not parental failure but systematic withdrawal of or failure to guarantee family support, forcing impossible choices on families while simultaneously portraying these placements as necessary and inevitable.

Human Rights Watch (HRW) (2017) has documented that medical professionals routinely encourage institutionalisation while discouraging alternatives. These professional judgements reflect deep-seated assumptions about which children belong in families and which can legitimately be segregated. Classification routinely marks certain children as 'uneducable' or 'untreatable' – labels that persist despite decades of evidence demonstrating all children's capacity to learn and develop. In Ukraine, researchers from Disability Rights International (DRI, 2022) encountered children with significant impairments categorised as having 'no prospects' and placed on trajectories of permanent institutionalisation. One institution director interviewed by DRI explicitly stated, 'Children who come here stay their whole life. This is their fate' (DRI, 2022, p 1). This fatalistic pronouncement reveals how classification operates not merely as description but as *prescription* – determining children's futures based on present-day evaluations of their perceived worth and potential.

The disposability of disabled children becomes particularly visible during crises. During the Russian invasion of Ukraine, DRI (2022) documented how children with the most significant impairments were left behind in dangerous regions, while non-disabled children or those with less visible impairments were evacuated to safety. It is difficult to imagine a starker example of how ableism as a *dispositif* of violence operates to determine whose lives are worth preserving and whose are expendable – some lives, it seems, are less grievable.

Examining the situation of young people with learning disabilities in Australian residential care, McCausland and Dowse (2022) identified a troubling transition – children's identities shift from being classified as 'at risk' to becoming perceived as 'a risk'. They observe that: 'The specific forms of surveillance and control they are subjected to mean that their designation of "at risk" almost routinely transmutes to "a risk" to others, to themselves, and to property' (McCausland and Dowse, 2022, p 8). This reclassification facilitates criminalisation rather than support, demonstrating how institutional logic transforms vulnerable children into threats that require containment. These processes operate across diverse contexts, but take on particular intensity at the intersections of multiple forms of marginalisation.

Within Canadian residential facilities, de Finney et al (2011) found that Indigenous youth experienced the intensified effects of institutional confinement through the intersection of disability with colonial histories and ongoing racism. The misinterpretation of their resistance as individual pathologies rather than as responses to systemic injustices and colonial histories (de Finney et al, 2011) reflects how intersecting systems of oppression shape institutional responses to multiply marginalised children.

Even when not formally incarcerated/institutionalised, disabled children all too often experience forms of 'soft confinement' through segregated educational placements, restrictive day programmes, or home confinement due to inadequate community support. These arrangements, while framed as necessary accommodations, often function as extensions of the carceral archipelago – limiting children's movement, social interaction, and development based on assumptions about their capabilities and needs.

The production of confinement thus operates through complex interactions between classification systems, resource constraints, cultural assumptions, and institutional imperatives. Rather than resulting from individual decisions or isolated factors, it emerges from those 'lines of force' within the *dispositif* that we have discussed – power relations that determine who can be confined, under what conditions, and with what justifications. These lines of force materialise through bureaucratic rationality (Bauman, 2004) – administrative systems that transform the management of 'human waste' from arbitrary cruelty to authorised intervention, rendering disabled children as objects to be 'processed' rather than subjects with rights.

Violence within the walls: applying the typology

> There were hundreds of people around me, but as a little boy, I didn't know another human being. Not properly. (Martin, 2019, p 3)

Once confined within institutional settings, disabled children experience various forms of violence that map directly onto our typology. These are not isolated incidents but patterned, predictable outcomes of the institutional environment itself – what Rossiter and Rinaldi (2018) term the 'violence continuum' inherent to institutional care.

Acts of commission

> If you were taken to Villa 5 at Kimberley, you knew you were in real trouble. The staff there were just evil. I saw this completely naked boy who had had an accident being hosed down by the staff using a fire hydrant hose. He would try to stand up and be knocked over again. I have seen many terrible things, but what I saw that day has stayed with me and still frightens me. It was a warning – if you misbehave, this will happen to you. (Martin, 2019, p 9)

Direct violence through acts of commission persists as an enduring feature of institutional environments worldwide. In Kazakhstan, one resident told HRW (2019, n.p.): 'They [staff] had a habit of beating us if we didn't want to help or if we didn't listen to them. They would also give us shots. Shots and shots of aminazine, to make us sleep'. This chemical restraint simultaneously subdues the body and silences protest. Children also experience other forms of restraint. One tragic case from Kazakhstan involved a seven-year-old child who 'died of asphyxiation after his caregiver reportedly tied him to his bed because he would not sleep and was disturbing other children' (HRW, 2019, n.p.).

In Germany, in 2010, a scandal erupted when staff at a residential care home for young disabled people were found to be verbally humiliating, withholding food, forcing the young people to sit on a chair for hours, using isolation practices, and several other forms of physical maltreatment (Lorenz, 2020). Elsewhere, HRW (2017) found that Greek institutions were confining children in caged beds due to staff shortages, while Indonesian facilities administered forced contraceptives to disabled girls without consent. In the UK, the Children's Commissioner's report *Unlocking Potential* (2015) found that disabled children in secure settings were 67% more likely than their non-disabled peers to experience isolation.

What Foucault termed the 'microphysics of power' (1991) manifests in these acts of commission. The institutional management of disabled children's bodies represents not merely the application of force but the use of disciplinary techniques aimed at producing compliant, manageable, docile subjects – normalised within broader regimes of truth that position disabled children's bodies as requiring control and 'rectification'.

Acts of omission

> I do not remember being picked up, or loved and cuddled, because there were so many of us, we were just a number. (Martin, 2019, p 2)

Perhaps more insidious are the harms that arise through inaction. In the UK, the death of Connor Sparrowhawk exemplifies this violence through omission. As previously described, despite his known epilepsy, Connor was left unsupervised by residential 'care' staff while taking a bath. Tragically, he drowned after having a seizure. The subsequent investigation found systematic failures in implementing appropriate observation protocols (Verita, 2014). Beyond the UK, Shannon et al's (2023) cross-national review across seven countries found that neglect of disabled children within institutional settings was particularly pervasive.

Physical, social and emotional neglect causes profound developmental harm. HRW (2017, n.p.) found that in Russian institutions, 'Children could not develop fully because of a lack of adequate nutrition and water'. In such circumstances, institutionalisation causes impairments in children who may not have had any pre-existing conditions. In Serbian facilities, they found medical neglect: 'a 15-year-old boy with untreated hydrocephalus, lying motionless on a bed' (HRW, 2016a, n.p.). In Ukraine, DRI (2022, p 4) has documented 'children and adolescents in bed during the day or tied up in a chair', desperate for social interaction and stimulus. Their investigators concluded that, for the children, this is 'painful, dangerous, and it is slowly killing them' (DRI, 2022, p 4). This observation captures omission as slow violence – harm that accumulates incrementally, its effects becoming visible only through developmental delays, physical deterioration, or psychological trauma.

Acts of commission by omission

> People who have power over other people are easily corrupted. Behind closed doors, the human rights of others are often violated. This should not be allowed, but it was allowed. (Martin, 2019, p 10)

Our typology's third category – commission by omission – captures deliberate decisions not to act despite awareness of needs and the capacity to address them. It usually involves the use of professional discretion. Returning to the case of Connor Sparrowhawk, the independent investigation into his death found that the unit where he was living operated under a 'business-as-usual' model despite *known* quality issues. This deliberate decision by managers to maintain inadequate care standards despite awareness of risks exemplifies commission by omission – knowledge of dangerous conditions coupled with decisions not to address them. Connor's tragic death also demonstrates how commission by omission operates through the *dispositif's* lines of force – institutional power relations that enable managers to maintain 'business-as-usual' standards despite awareness of deadly risks. These lines of force intersect with lines of utterance that frame such decisions as 'professional judgement' rather than deliberate endangerment.

Elsewhere, despite clear evidence that family connections improve outcomes, institutions across contexts deliberately restrict family visits, communication channels, and community participation, actively severing ties that might provide both emotional support and potential pathways out of confinement (HRW, 2019). Further, HRW (2019) has documented practices of deliberate denial of communication and rehabilitation support to disabled children. This failure to provide alternative communication methods to children in institutions is a problem around the world and reflects assumptions that certain forms of communication are dispensable and certain voices superfluous.

Acts of omission by commission

> Everyone has a right to a life instead of wasting away in institutions waiting to die. That is not a life. (Martin, 2019, p 26)

Our final typology category – omission by commission – reveals how formal policies systematically withdraw protection from disabled children through the deliberate removal of safeguards. Connor Sparrowhawk's case demonstrated this through what investigators identified as systematic withdrawal of protection through inadequate policy frameworks – specifically no statutory learning disability framework and no enforceable national standards for units, such as the short-term assessment and treatment unit where Connor was staying (Verita, 2014, 2015). These gaps reflect deliberate policy decisions that leave institutionalised disabled people with fewer safeguards.

Further, this violence manifests clearly in funding models that favour institutions over community care. For example, in a policy choice clearly not driven by lack of resources, Guatemala spends 45 times more to institutionalise children than to support family-based care (DRI and Colectivo Vida Independiente, 2018). Shannon et al's (2023) cross-national review reveals that the Guatemala situation is not an anomaly – family support systems are being systematically undermined in many countries, both in majority and minority worlds.

Legal frameworks facilitating minimally overseen institutionalisation constitute another serious form of this violence. A pattern documented globally by the UN CRPD Committee shows that disabled children are routinely placed in institutions with less scrutiny than their non-disabled peers. In Kazakhstan, placement in residential institutions remains the first response for children with disabilities, while children without disabilities are more likely to be placed in family-type settings (HRW 2019, UNICEF 2025). HRW (2017) confirms that in many countries, disability alone is sufficient justification for institutionalization. Children are placed in institutions without any judicial oversight.

Deinstitutionalisation and its discontents: the mutation of carceral logics

> I feel in lots of ways we have just swapped large institutions for smaller ones. Residential group homes have different bricks, but it is the thoughts, feelings, and actions of others that make a place an institution. (Martin, 2019, p 26)

By applying our typology to institutional settings, we see violence against disabled children not as an aberration but as intrinsic to ableism's carceral manifestation – a *dispositif* of violence operating through direct action, neglect, deliberate inaction, and systematic protection withdrawal. But what of the move towards deinstitutionalisation? Over the past six decades, deinstitutionalisation movements have achieved significant reductions in the number of disabled people confined to large facilities. Countries across the minority world have closed many of their historic asylums, long-stay hospitals, and residential schools. Yet these apparent successes often mask a more troubling reality – deinstitutionalisation has frequently reconfigured rather than dismantled carceral logics, shifting the sites and forms of confinement without necessarily challenging its underlying rationalities (Ben-Moshe, 2020).

This reconfiguration aligns with what Series (2022) terms the 'post-carceral' landscape of care – a terrain in which institutional logics have migrated into community-based services, domestic spaces, and legal frameworks. Series (2022, p 6), who draws extensively on the work of Ben-Moshe (2020), observes that 'community care has been described as part of a broader "institutional archipelago" (…) a carceral "continuum" extending from traditional sites of detention (…) out into community settings'. Her analysis shows how disciplinary power spreads beyond formal institutions to permeate seemingly non-institutional spaces.

This persistence of institutional logics despite physical changes reveals how the *dispositif's* lines adapt rather than disappear. *Lines of visibility* shift to render small-scale settings invisible as 'institutions' while maintaining many of the features of institutionalisation. *Lines of utterance* reframe segregation as 'specialised care' or 'family-like' provision. *Lines of force* migrate from large institutional hierarchies to professionalised 'care relationships' that maintain similar power imbalances. *Lines of subjectivation* continue producing disabled subjects as requiring containment, merely in smaller, more dispersed sites.

In the UK context, Connor Sparrowhawk's death illuminates this post-carceral landscape. Despite occurring in a small, community-based assessment unit rather than a traditional institution, Connor's death revealed how the same carceral logics – the devaluation of disabled lives, the prioritisation of professional knowledge, and systematic withdrawal of protection – operate across the social care archipelago. The *#Justice4LB* campaign, following Connor's death, challenged not only specific failures of care at the unit where he died, but also the broader system that endangers the lives of disabled people. Connor's mother, Sara Ryan's (2017) powerful memoir, *Justice for Laughing Boy,* documents this struggle in compelling detail.

The unit where Connor lived and died is one of a number of smaller residential facilities that have come to replace larger institutions for children and young people globally. Another type is the group home. The UN CRPD Committee (2017) has explicitly rejected the notion that small group homes are fundamentally different from institutions. Evidence from multiple countries supports this position (see Beckett, 2021, for a summary of evidence). DRI (2013) documented that children with disabilities in Bulgarian small group homes were living lives of isolation and neglect, exposed to violence, sexual abuse, and bullying. Fylkesnes' (2021) ethnographic research in Norwegian group homes found that they maintained hierarchical relationships, surveillance practices, and staff-centred routines despite their small scale. Staff frequently talked about children over their heads, using institutional codes that reinforced their status as objects rather than subjects. One staff member explicitly stated, 'We are not their parents' (Fylkesnes, 2021, p 1007) – a declaration marking the boundaries of professional care within these supposedly home-like environments. As Beckett (2021, p 3) argues, 'family-like institutions are still institutions' regardless of size, and the 'family-like fiction masks non-familial realities'.

This persistence of institutions and institutional logics reveals the distinction Ben-Moshe (2020) makes between reform and abolition. Most deinstitutionalisation efforts merely relocate or improve conditions without challenging fundamental assumptions about segregation. Without confronting ableism as a *dispositif* of violence that constructs certain children as requiring confinement, these reforms reconfigure rather than dismantle institutionalisation. Abolition requires not just facility closures but entirely new ways of understanding, valuing, and supporting disabled lives.

Resistance and complex personhood

> I told her, 'No. You are not my mum.' She slapped me in the face. I told her to 'f off.' She kicked me, and then I kicked her back. I had been abused for years, and I had had a gutsful. (Martin, 2019, p 16)

Empirical research consistently documents that disabled children and young people are not passive victims of confinement – they resist, adapt, subvert, and transform the spaces they are forced to inhabit. Earlier in this chapter, we mentioned that de Finney et al (2011) found that Indigenous youth in Canadian residential facilities employ strategic resistance tactics, such as verbal defiance, refusal to participate in mandated activities, silence, and strategic compliance. More recently, McCausland and Dowse (2022) found that young people with learning disabilities living in Australian residential care settings actively and creatively resisted oppressive conditions. Understanding this resistance is crucial for recognising complex personhood – the full humanity of institutionalised people beyond reductive narratives of victimhood or pathology. These resistance practices embody Foucault's (1998, p 95) insight that 'where there is power, there is resistance'. Resistance never operates from outside power networks but within them, using their strategic possibilities against dominating intent. When a child creates meaning within an institutional space designed to nullify it or forms relationships exceeding institutional boundaries, they engage in what Foucault terms 'counter-conduct' – contesting power relations while navigating their constraints. These acts of resistance also represent what Deleuze and Guattari (2004) terms 'lines of flight' – vectors that escape or redirect the *dispositif's* established patterns of visibility, utterance, force, and subjectivation, creating alternative possibilities for disabled children's becoming and creative transformation.

The situation is, however, complex. In both cases mentioned above (Canada and Australia), staff frequently interpreted children's expressions of resistance as 'challenging behaviours' or criminal actions (de Finney et al, 2011; McCausland and Dowse, 2022). Institutional systems thus refuse to acknowledge children's agency, instead interpreting legitimate expressions of dissent as further evidence of pathology requiring control.

This reveals the particular constraints to resistance within institutional settings for children. Confinement creates a sophisticated form of capture where the very act of resistance becomes reframed as confirmation of the need for continued containment. The spatial confinement, surveillance practices, and professional authority combine to suspend normal expectations of autonomy and rights. This capture operates with particular intensity for disabled children, whose resistance encounters both ableist and ageist frameworks that deny their capacity for legitimate dissent. Opposition becomes transformed into symptom, challenge into pathology – a circular logic that renders institutional control seemingly inevitable while concealing its violence.

Beyond the acts of disabled children and youth, their families also forge their own resistance pathways. Despite the systematic devaluation of their knowledge and expertise, many parents maintain persistent advocacy for their institutionalised children. They challenge treatment decisions. They demand inclusion in care planning. They refuse institutional inevitability. HRW (2016b) documented parents like Jasmina Čuković in Serbia who actively resisted medical pressure to institutionalise their children, advocating instead for community-based support despite professional discouragement.

Connor Sparrowhawk's death catalysed perhaps the most visible example of collaborative resistance in the UK context. The *#Justice4LB* campaign brought together Connor's family, disability activists, academics, and other allies. Led by his mother, Sara Ryan, and stepfather, Richard Huggins, the campaign deployed social media, legal challenges, artivism, and community organising to demand accountability and system change (Ryan, 2017). This activism contested not only the specific failures in Connor's care but also the broader devaluation of disabled lives within care systems – making the violence visible when institutions worked to conceal it.

Yet again, however, there is often push-back. Ryan (2017) powerfully describes how she was called 'toxic' by a medical professional working at the unit where her son Connor died because she questioned the quality of his care. This labelling exemplifies how institutions reframe family advocacy as problematic interference, pathologising resistance itself when it threatens institutional authority.

Resistance to institutionalisation thus requires not only practical alternatives to confinement but epistemological alternatives to the ableist frameworks that produce certain children as requiring segregation and *a determination not to be silenced*. It demands what Ben-Moshe terms 'abolition as knowledge and ways of unknowing' (2020, p 111) – the dismantling of certainties about who belongs where and what constitutes appropriate care. Disabled children and their families are challenging not just specific institutions but the entire knowledge system that renders some bodies and minds as inherently requiring containment and control – and they need others to rally behind and with them. By centring the complex personhood of institutionalised children and amplifying their acts of resistance alongside family advocacy, we can begin to envision care practices that honour rather than suppress resistance, and communities that embrace and affirm difference rather than confine it to the margins of society.

Conclusion

> My life in institutions meant I personally had nothing and no one to call my own. I learnt that I was somehow a nobody – that my life didn't really matter. (Martin, 2019, p 23)

Throughout this chapter, we have analysed the confinement of disabled children and youth as a manifestation of ableism, functioning as a *dispositif* of violence. By examining how institutions operate as sites where multiple forms of violence converge, we have demonstrated the nature of institutional harm. This is not a matter of isolated incidents but a structured system that produces certain children as requiring segregation, surveillance, and control.

Our analysis has applied the typology of violence that we developed in Chapter 2 – commission, omission, commission by omission, and omission by commission – to institutional settings, revealing how violence operates through direct action, neglect, deliberate and permitted inaction, and the systematic withdrawal of protection. These forms are not aberrations but constitutive elements of institutional care itself, reflecting broader ableist logics that devalue disabled children's lives.

Connor Sparrowhawk's preventable death in a supposedly therapeutic setting shows how ableism functions as a *dispositif* of violence through multiple mechanisms. His story reveals epistemic violence in the devaluation of family knowledge, violence through omission in inadequate supervision, commission by omission in the decision to maintain inadequate care standards, and omission by commission in the systemic withdrawal of protection through inadequate policy frameworks. The *#Justice4LB* campaign exemplifies resistance to institutional violence, challenging not only specific failures but the broader system that positions disabled lives as less valuable. For those in the UK Disability Studies community, this case continues to resonate as a powerful reminder of both institutional failure and the possibilities for collective resistance.

Our analysis of Connor's case and institutional practices more broadly revealed how ableism as a *dispositif* of violence operates through the four lines identified in Chapter 3. *Lines of visibility* determined which aspects of Connor's needs were seen while rendering family knowledge invisible; *lines of utterance* privileged medical discourse over experiential expertise; *lines of force* enabled institutional authority to override family concerns; and *lines of subjectivation* positioned Connor within deficit categories rather than recognising his full personhood. These same lines operate across the institutional archipelago, adapting to new settings while maintaining their fundamental function of containing and controlling disabled lives.

Drawing on Foucault's theorisation of disciplinary power, we have shown how institutions operate as technologies of normalisation and control, producing 'docile bodies' through techniques of classification, surveillance, and correction. Series' (2022) analysis of the post-carceral landscape of care has illuminated how institutional logics have migrated beyond traditional sites of confinement. Her observation that 'the socio-legal landscape of care is haunted by its carceral past' (Series, 2022, p 1) captures, so poignantly, how contemporary approaches to disability support continue to operate through mechanisms of control despite rhetorics of inclusion.

We have examined how deinstitutionalisation has often reconfigured rather than dismantled carceral logics – shifting the sites and forms of confinement without challenging underlying rationalities. This explains why, despite decades of reform, institutionalisation persists as a response to childhood disability, mutating into new forms while maintaining its function of containing disabled bodies and minds.

Crucially, we have also examined resistance to institutionalisation – how disabled children, their families, and advocates challenge and transform spaces of confinement. The resistance of disabled children reflects their complex personhood – the fact that they can and do maintain dignity, creativity/becoming and humanity, despite systems designed to deny these qualities. Yet institutional settings create particular constraints on resistance, where children's expressions of dissent are systematically reframed as pathology, while family advocacy is dismissed as 'toxic' interference that threatens professional authority.

As we move to Chapter 6 on assisted dying and terminalism, this analysis provides essential context for understanding how ableism operates across diverse domains. The classificatory systems marking certain children as requiring institutional management connect directly to evaluative frameworks determining which lives are worth preserving. The professional authorities justifying segregation employ similar logics to those framing assisted dying as a compassionate choice. The funding models prioritising institutional over community-based support reflect the same economic rationalities influencing end-of-life decisions.

Most fundamentally, both institutionalisation and assisted dying emerge from what we identified in Chapter 2 as 'social death' – the process through which certain individuals are deemed to have 'lives not worth living' *before* biological death. The institutional declaration: 'Children who come here stay their whole life. This is their fate' reflects the same logic underlying assisted dying regimes, where disabled lives are constructed as inherently burdensome or tragic. Both operate through 'differential grievability', determining whose lives are deemed worthy of protection and whose can be contained, limited, or ended.

By recognising these connections, we better understand how different manifestations of ableism, functioning as a *dispositif* of violence, operate not as isolated phenomena but as interconnected elements of a broader system. This understanding informs more effective strategies for resistance, addressing not only specific forms of violence but the underlying *dispositif* that enables and sustains them.

Cutaway 4: Deinstitutionalisation and group homes

In 2021, Angharad E. Beckett made a submission to the United Nations Committee on the Rights of the Child regarding their General Day of Discussion on Alternative Care, addressing concerns about group homes for disabled children.

Miro: Angharad, what motivated your submission to the UN Committee about group homes?

Angharad: I became concerned about the direction of policy discourse. There's been this push toward 'group homes' as supposedly being better alternatives to large institutions. While I support deinstitutionalisation, I was troubled by what appeared to me to be a case of creating smaller institutions with a different name.

Miro: That ambiguity seems problematic. How are 'group homes' being defined?

Angharad: There's no universally agreed definition, which creates a fuzzy controversy. Some describe settings with just a few children. Others include facilities housing up to 40 children! Alternative terms like 'small family homes' or 'family-like care' appear across policy documents, but it's unclear whether these describe the same thing. Even the *Lancet Commission on Institutionalisation and Deinstitutionalisation* seemed confused. They classified group homes as institutions in one publication, then distinguished them from institutional care in another published the same month!

Miro: Yes, I've often heard these places described as being like a family home. What did your review of international research reveal about this claim?

Angharad: What makes a family, or a sense of home, is fundamentally emotional. 'Family', at best, is associated with a feeling of belonging, and 'home' with where we feel safe and can exert control over our environment. That sense of control creates the foundation for genuine relationships. Small group homes consistently fail to provide these elements. Staff rotate on shifts – parents might share responsibilities for care, but they are never 'off duty'! There are regulations, lack of privacy. Group homes remain institutions, despite the change in terminology.

Miro: Were there methodological issues with the evidence supporting group homes?

Angharad: I identified two particularly problematic patterns in the evidence being employed to support group homes. First, much research is conducted by or funded by organisations that run group homes, which raises questions about what research methodologists call 'funding effect' or 'sponsorship effect'.

Miro: That sounds a bit dodgy to me!

Angharad: Indeed! Second, there is a privileging of research from medical and psychological sciences. These studies focus on quantifiable indicators like standardised tests or measures like head circumference to determine whether children living in group homes (or other institutions) are experiencing adverse effects. They rarely, if ever, seek the children's opinions. There's a form of 'scientism' at work, I think. A narrow range of research designs is considered 'credible', predominantly quantitative measures that tell us little about children's experiences or aspirations.

Miro: What does the evidence tell us about outcomes for children in group homes?

Angharad: There's remarkably little evidence showing unequivocally positive outcomes. Even studies that find generally positive results note concerning issues regarding children's educational achievement or involvement with criminal justice systems in later life. We see recurring concerns about group homes, such as harsh punishments, limited family contact, the use of restraints, and violations of privacy and dignity. The geographical spread of evidence is telling – from Bulgaria to Botswana, from Serbia to Norway.

Miro: If group homes aren't the answer, what is?

Angharad: We need to address two fundamental questions often overlooked in debates about alternative care: Why are so many disabled children in alternative care to begin with? And why are disabled children deemed 'hard to place' in adoption or foster care? Research consistently shows that poverty and inadequate support services create crises for families. Evidence from Sweden, for example, documents parents experiencing exhaustion due to insufficient support. But there are early intervention programmes that demonstrate that families can be effectively supported to stay together – and importantly, there is good practice happening in low-resource contexts, so insufficient funding is clearly not a barrier.

Miro: You've mentioned some promising alternatives. What specific approaches show promise?

Angharad: Programmes like REPARE (Reasonable Efforts to Permanency Through Adoption and Reunification Endeavors) in the US have been particularly effective. Rather than removing children, they empower families through ecological development approaches. The *Getting to Know Cerebral Palsy* programme offers parent training and peer support networks in many countries in the Majority and Minority world. In Nepal, multi-faceted initiatives combining healthcare improvements, sign language training for parents, and microfinance support have shown remarkable success in keeping families together.

For children who genuinely require alternative care, we must challenge the professional pessimism around placing disabled children with families. This pessimism becomes a self-fulfilling prophecy, but research shows it's unwarranted. With appropriate policies and practices, disabled children can thrive in genuine family environments rather than institutions, regardless of how small or rebranded they might be.

If you'd like to read Angharad's full submission to the UN Convention on the Rights of the Child (CRC) Committee, it can be found here: https://www.ohchr.org/sites/default/files/documents/hrbodies/crc/discussions/2021/submissions/subm-2021-day-general-aca-angharad-beckett-university-leeds.pdf [Accessed: 20 September 2025].

6

Assisted dying and terminalism

Our analysis thus far has examined the manifestation of ableism as a *dispositif* through interpersonal violence and microaggressions (Chapter 4) and confinement (Chapter 5). In this chapter, we turn to what is perhaps the most profound manifestation of ableism as a *dispositif* of violence – assisted dying and terminalism.

We recognise that the issues discussed in this chapter are deeply painful for many people on either side of the debate. This pain, whether experienced by those advocating for assisted dying or those opposing it, deserves acknowledgement. Nevertheless, we must be open about our political positioning – we are fundamentally opposed to assisted dying. Indeed, Miro Griffiths, co-author of this book, is a leading member of the *Not Dead Yet Campaign* in the UK, which actively opposes assisted dying legislation.

We recognise that assisted dying debates within Disability Studies are not monolithic. Shakespeare (2022) supports assisted dying narrowly limited to terminal illness, while explicitly warning against extension to those with long-term impairments due to the risk that a decision might be due to inadequate social support. By contrast, Ouellette (2017) approaches the issue through disability equality, arguing that where assisted dying laws exist, they must not create discriminatory barriers that deny disabled people equal access. Clearly these authors' interventions differ. What neither offers, however, is a sufficiently robust critique of the fundamental logic of assisted dying and the frameworks that systematically construct disability as grounds for considering death. It is this robust critique that we strive to present herein.

We follow others in the field of bioethics (see Sumner, 2011, for useful discussion) in understanding assisted dying to include both 'active' and 'passive' euthanasia. Active euthanasia involves directly administering lethal substances, while passive euthanasia involves withholding or withdrawing life-sustaining treatment. We engage with the concept of 'terminalism' – a form of discrimination that extends beyond those who are actually dying. Reed (2024, p 108) defines terminalism as 'discrimination against the dying or treating the terminally ill worse than they would expect to be treated if they were not dying'. Importantly, he identifies that this discrimination extends to those who are not imminently dying. As Reed (2024) clarifies, membership in this socially salient group includes those where terminal illness is understood in relation to prognosis rather than immediate death. This conceptualisation encompasses situations where individuals are denied treatment or support based on quality-of-life assessments or because their conditions are deemed life-limiting, even when death is not imminent.

It is important to clarify the relationship between terminalism and ableism, which overlap but are not identical. Both contribute to systems that marginalise individuals based on perceived vulnerability or lack of productivity, but they operate with different targets and foci. Terminalism specifically targets the dying or those categorised as having a terminal illness, while ableism targets all disabled people, regardless of their prognosis. Similarly, terminalism often focuses on end-of-life care and medical decisions, while ableism encompasses a broader range of social and systemic issues. Nevertheless, both operate through parallel logics of devaluation and contribute to the same *dispositif* of violence.

Han (2024) explains how terminalism operates through institutional medical knowledge. Terminally ill patients, notably in ICUs, problematise and challenge medicine's distinction between dead and living bodies. 'Medicine discursively disciplines the dying to fit into its conceptual framework; the dying are understood as "broken machines" without value' (Han 2024, p 116). Reed (2024) identifies allocation protocols for scarce medical resources as an example of terminalism. Such protocols demonstrate how healthcare systems withdraw support from those categorised as having limited futures.

While ableism devalues disabled lives based on perceived deviation from normative functioning, terminalism extends this devaluation to those who are dying or perceived to be dying – or indeed, anyone categorised with an illness that is likely to eventually lead to their death, even when their death is unlikely to occur soon. Terminalism reproduces ableist assumptions about what constitutes a 'worthwhile life' – one that not only aligns with normative functioning but also has a certain temporality, extending into a 'viable future' where it is possible to imagine someone contributing 'meaningfully' to society.

The expansion of assisted dying legislation globally has been rapid and concerning. Assisted dying has now been legalised in multiple countries and subnational jurisdictions worldwide, and in many of these contexts, the trajectory shows expansion beyond original parameters. While initial assisted dying frameworks typically focused on terminal illness, many jurisdictions have seen expansion beyond this, although this pattern is not universal.

For example, in Oregon, despite formal legislative stability, Finegan (2024) documents significant empirical slippage: assisted deaths increased tenfold from 16 in 1998 to 278 in 2022, with evidence of diagnostic drift toward less clearly terminal conditions and acceptance of 'burden-based' motivations that were originally rejected. This pattern demonstrates how expansion can occur through clinical interpretation and administrative modifications even without legislative change, while formal restrictions on residency requirements and waiting periods have also been reduced (Oregon Health Authority, 2023).

In this chapter, we do not engage with traditional ethical debates about autonomy versus protection. Rather, we seek to reframe assisted dying and terminalism as manifestations of ableism as a *dispositif* of violence – examining how they operate within broader networks of power, knowledge, and materiality to devalue and eliminate certain forms of bodily and cognitive difference. We argue that assisted dying practices and discourses cannot be understood in isolation from the socio-political contexts that render some lives less grievable (Butler, 2004) and more disposable (Mbembe, 2003) than others. Our analysis will demonstrate that what presents as individual choice is systematically shaped by societal structures and attitudes that construct disability as inherently tragic, burdensome, and less worthy of life-sustaining investment.

To understand assisted dying as a manifestation of ableism, as a *dispositif* of violence, we must examine how it operates through its four lines (as introduced in Chapter 3). *Lines of visibility* determine which bodies become seen as legitimate candidates for death, rendering certain impairments as markers of lives 'not worth living'. *Lines of utterance* establish medical and bioethical discourses that frame death as a compassionate choice while marginalising disabled people's own knowledge about living with impairment. *Lines of force* manifest through clinical authority that can propose death as 'treatment' while withholding alternative supports. *Lines of subjectivation* shape how disabled people come to understand themselves within frameworks that position their lives as burdensome rather than valued.

Necropolitics, thanatopolitics, and biopower

To understand assisted dying and terminalism as manifestations of ableism, we must situate them within broader theoretical frameworks of power and governance. Foucault's (1998) concept of biopower – the regulation and optimisation of life at the population level – provides our starting point. Biopower represents a shift from sovereign power's right to 'take life or let live' toward modern governance's power to 'foster life or disallow it to the point of death' (Foucault, 1998, p 138). This transition reconfigures death's centrality within new relations of power.

Mbembe (2003, p 11) extends this analysis through necropolitics, defined as the deployment of sovereign power to determine 'who may live and who must die'. This framework illuminates how assisted dying operates through decisions regarding which lives warrant preservation and which might legitimately be ended. Within Disability Studies, Grue (2022) further develops these concepts through thanatopolitics – governance related specifically to death. Unlike earlier authoritarian forms that imposed death directly, contemporary neoliberal thanatopolitics operates indirectly, presenting death as a choice, right, or responsibility. This mirrors broader governance trends emphasising individual autonomy while obscuring structural conditions that constrain 'choice'. Neoliberal thanatopolitical discourses operate through what Grue (2022, n.p.) terms 'parrhesiastic rhetoric' – truth-telling from positions of vulnerability that lends assisted dying authenticity and legitimacy. This rhetorical operation masks how structural conditions, such as poverty, inadequate healthcare, or lack of support, shape decisions to pursue assisted dying.

We find that Bishop's (2016) work on the 'anticipatory corpse' allows us to understand how modern medicine's epistemological foundation predisposes it toward thanatopolitical practices. His analysis shows how medicine's corpse-centred epistemology reduces living bodies to mechanistic systems evaluated by their proximity to normative functioning. When combined with neoliberal economic rationalities, the result creates a context where bodies deemed too deviant from norms become candidates for elimination rather than support.

The global expansion of assisted dying: a slippery slope realised

Proponents of assisted dying have typically argued that carefully crafted legislation with strict safeguards can prevent abuse and protect vulnerable populations. Examining the trajectory of assisted dying in jurisdictions where it has been legalised reveals a consistent pattern of expansion beyond initial boundaries – what is colloquially called the 'slippery slope'. This term is sometimes dismissed as a fallacious argument, but empirical evidence demonstrates that it accurately describes what happens when assisted dying is legalised (Tremain, 2019; Coelho et al, 2023; Colleran and Doherty, 2024). Since implementing Medical Assistance in Dying (MAID) in 2016, Canada has seen substantial increases in assisted deaths. According to Health Canada's Annual Report on Medical Assistance in Dying 2023, MAID accounted for 4.7% of all Canadian deaths in 2023, with the most significant expansion occurring in 2021 when the 'reasonably foreseeable death' requirement was removed (Health Canada, 2024).

Even more concerning than the numbers (which are alarming) is the progressive expansion of eligibility criteria, with the removal of the 'reasonably foreseeable death' requirement in 2021 opening MAID to people with chronic conditions and impairments who are not terminally ill (Health Canada, 2022). This expansion has led to documented cases where MAID has functioned as a response to social and economic problems rather than terminal illness (Ministry of the Solicitor General, Office of the Chief Coroner, 2024). MAID appears to be serving as a de facto solution to suffering caused by poverty, loneliness, inadequate housing, and poor care services – issues that should be alleviated via social policy responses (Cheng, 2023).

Similar patterns of expansion are evident in other jurisdictions. In Belgium, one of four countries where assisted suicide for children is legal, there is no minimum age requirement if children are 'deemed competent' (Raus, 2016). In Colombia, following the legalisation of euthanasia for terminal patients in 1997, the Constitutional Court extended eligibility to non-terminal patients in 2021, marking a significant expansion beyond initial parameters (World Federation of Right to Die Societies, 2021). Elsewhere, assisted suicide is being permitted on the grounds of psychosocial impairments, including eating disorders. Roff and Cook-Cottone (2024, p 1) document at least 60 known cases of assisted death for patients diagnosed with eating disorders across multiple jurisdictions, noting that 'clinical rationales used to affirm patients with the condition were eligible for assisted death lack validity and do not cohere with empirical understanding'. Their research reveals that 100% of patients who received assisted death for eating disorders were women, highlighting intersectional dimensions that have yet to be addressed (Roff and Cook-Cottone, 2024).

The concepts of 'intolerable suffering' and 'irremediability' – key eligibility criteria in many jurisdictions – have proven particularly problematic. There is evidence of substantial subjectivity in assessment, with clinicians sometimes accepting patient claims of intolerable suffering at face value without objective measures or attempts at amelioration. While we are *not* suggesting that the feelings of patients be disregarded or dismissed, there are real dangers with this approach. As Maung (2023) argues, suffering arises not merely from internal states but from the interaction between individuals and their social–environmental contexts. Suffering deemed 'intolerable' often reflects inadequate support systems, discrimination, poverty, and social isolation rather than inherent features of impairment or illness.

We are concerned that the global expansion of assisted dying reveals the operation of what Foucault (1991, 1998) would likely describe as a strategy without a strategist – a coherent direction of development that emerges from interconnected discourses, institutions, and practices without requiring explicit coordination. Examining assisted dying through our *dispositif* framework reveals how it operates through interconnected lines that constitute ableism as a system of violence. *Lines of visibility* that determine which bodies become visible as candidates for assisted death, with disability functioning as a marker that makes certain lives appear as 'strong candidates'. *Lines of utterance* that govern what can be said about suffering and quality of life, with medical and bioethical discourses rendering certain forms of embodiment as inherently burdensome (on oneself and others). *Lines of force* that manifest in the power dynamics between medical professionals and disabled people, where discretionary authority allows for professionals to propose death as a 'solution' to disablement. *Lines of subjectivation* that shape how disabled people come to understand themselves within ableist and terminalist frameworks, potentially internalising the notion that their lives represent burdens rather than valued existences. These interconnected lines demonstrate how assisted dying operates not as an isolated practice but as part of ableism as a *dispositif* of violence.

Terminalism and ableism: analysing forms of violence

Building on our typology developed in Chapter 2, we now examine how assisted dying and terminalism operate through four interrelated forms of violence. Doing so allows us to understand the complex and multifaceted ways in which ableism as violence devalues and eliminates disabled lives.

Acts of commission: the direct provision of death

The most visible form of violence within assisted dying frameworks is the act of commission through *active euthanasia* – the direct provision of lethal drugs. In jurisdictions such as Canada, Belgium, and the Netherlands, the direct provision of death through euthanasia constitutes a medical act performed by healthcare professionals. This medicalisation of death transforms killing into treatment, obscuring its nature as an act of violence. As Bishop (2016) observes, medical authorities in many countries already participate directly in deciding who is eligible for healthcare – acting as gatekeepers. When these authorities also decide who should be offered death, the power imbalance becomes profound.

The commission of assisted death becomes particularly problematic when applied to disabled people whose conditions are not terminal. While initial assisted dying frameworks typically focused on terminal illness, their expansion to include chronic conditions, non-life-threatening impairments, and mental illness reflects what Mbembe (2003, p 17) identifies as the 'distribution of death' across populations deemed less valuable. When patients with conditions like spinal cord injuries, autism, or psychiatric diagnoses receive assisted death, as documented in Canada and elsewhere (Lemmens, 2023), this reflects how ableism creates the conditions that lead to such requests. The suffering that drives people to seek death frequently stems from social and environmental factors, such as failures in care, institutionalisation, inaccessible environments, and a lack of neuro-inclusive practices. As the case of Larry McAfee demonstrates (discussed on the following pages), when appropriate support becomes available, the desire to die can completely disappear. While we do not discount that some suffering may be directly related to medical conditions, there is strong evidence that many requests are motivated by distress and despair in the face of societal failures, rather than physical pain or medical symptoms alone.

Understanding how violence operates through assisted dying requires examining not only active euthanasia but also how systems respond to requests for treatment withdrawal. Longmore's (2003) analysis of two high-profile cases in the USA – those of David Rivlin and Larry McAfee – provides crucial historical context. Both men, quadriplegic ventilator users, sought to discontinue life-sustaining treatment primarily due to social isolation, institutionalisation, and a lack of social care in their communities. These early cases from the 1980s and 1990s established troubling precedents in which courts interpreted requests for death from disabled people primarily through the lens of individual autonomy while systematically overlooking social and institutional factors.

As Longmore (2003) convincingly argues, the non-disabled people around both men articulated their decision as being logical – a type of rational suicide – despite clear evidence that their suffering stemmed primarily from institutionalisation and inadequate support services. This framing reveals the epistemological implications of ableism, whereby certain thoughts and reasoning processes are positioned as inherently 'logical' or 'rational' when they align with ableist assumptions. Significantly, when Mr McAfee later received appropriate support services, he withdrew his request to die:

> But something unexpected happened. People from United Cerebral Palsy offered Larry McAfee creative possibilities to regain control of his life and to work in computer engineering, and he changed his mind about dying. In fact, he ended up testifying before the Georgia state legislature, calling upon them to fund independent living. He told them that if it had been available, he would not have despaired to the point of seeking death. (Longmore, 2003, p 184)

Mr McAfee's transformation demonstrates how the 'choice' of death can be shaped by social conditions rather than inherent suffering from impairment. His case reveals that assisted dying offers an individual-level, biological solution to what is, so often, a social, institutional, and material problem – constituting a form of violence that targets the victims of social injustice rather than confronting the injustice itself.

Acts of omission: the failure to provide alternatives

Acts of omission within assisted dying contexts involve the failure to provide adequate alternatives to death. These include inadequate palliative care, insufficient disability support services, lack of accessible housing, poverty reduction measures, and mental health services. When people choose assisted death because better options are unavailable, this constitutes violence through omission.

In Colombia, which has had legal euthanasia since 1997, research reveals that access to palliative care remains 'very deficient' and 'mostly concentrated in larger cities' (de Vries et al, 2021, n.p.). This inadequate provision of care alternatives occurs alongside concerning practices, including cases where patients received drugs 'with the explicit intention to hasten death without their explicit request' (de Vries et al, 2021, n.p.) and pervasive failures in communication between doctors and patients about end-of-life decisions. When people experiencing extreme pain or distress lack access to adequate palliative care, the choice of death is, we contend, a reflection of systemic healthcare failures.

These omissions reflect what Sallnow et al (2025, p 104) identify when they note that '(a)ssisted dying could be seen as easier and cheaper than building health equity' and ensuring good palliative care. The failure to provide adequate alternatives represents a systematic devaluation of certain lives. This form of violence operates more subtly than direct commission but can be equally deadly.

Commission by omission: the deliberate withholding of support

Commission by omission involves deliberate decisions by professionals with discretionary authority to withhold necessary support or intervention despite awareness of need and the technical ability to act. In the context of assisted dying, this typically manifests as withholding medical treatments, social supports, or accommodations from disabled or chronically ill people while simultaneously offering assisted death as an alternative. The case of Canadian veteran Christine Gauthier exemplifies this form of violence. When Ms Gauthier requested a stairlift for her home, a Veterans Affairs caseworker suggested MAID instead (Hurley, 2022). This was not mere negligence but a deliberate decision to offer death rather than accommodation.

Another well-known case is that of Roger Foley, who lives in Canada. Mr Foley has a neurological condition causing physical impairment (Stainton, 2023). He recorded hospital staff repeatedly offering him MAID while denying his requests for self-directed home care (recordings available at https://assistedlab.ch/audio/roger-foley-s-audio-recordings, accessed April 2025). Foley made these recordings public to expose the pressure he faced – showing how inadequate social support, combined with an offer of assisted death, created a coercive environment. Foley's resistance to MAID represents not merely a personal struggle but also his opposition to a system positioning death as an 'acceptable' response to disability-related needs. His case demonstrates how seemingly compassionate offers of the 'choice' of death mask the systemic devaluation of disabled lives and function as sophisticated forms of violence.

This pattern of deliberately withholding support extends beyond formal MAID frameworks to broader medical decision-making through *passive euthanasia*. An ongoing legal case illustrates this issue (for further discussion, see Chapters 2 and 7). Michael Hickson, a quadriplegic African American man, was denied intensive care for COVID-19 due to quality-of-life assessments that, it would seem, deemed his life not worth saving. Such cases demonstrate how the same ableist logics operate whether through active provision of death or withdrawal of life-sustaining treatment.

Further, the complexity and reality of coercion by others in assisted dying contexts is extensively documented by Colleran and Doherty (2024). They note reports include patients 'pressurised to EAS' (euthanasia and assisted suicide) by family members, undermining the voluntary basis of these decisions (Colleran and Doherty, 2024, p 358).

While determining if coercion is involved is difficult, when healthcare professionals are aware of such pressures yet proceed with assisted dying anyway or *fail to adequately investigate potential coercion,* then we argue that this also represents violence through commission by omission – a deliberate non-intervention that results in death.

Omission by commission: systematic removal of protections

The final form of violence in our typology is omission by commission – the systematic removal of protections through explicit policy decisions or legislative changes. In the context of assisted dying, this operates through multiple but interconnected rationalities that converge on making death more accessible while reducing safeguards for vulnerable populations.

One mechanism operates through a rights-expansion logic that extends assisted dying to new populations. When Canada removed the 'reasonably foreseeable death' requirement from MAID legislation in 2021, it systematically withdrew protection from people with chronic conditions and disabled people under the banner of equality – arguing that non-terminal conditions should not exclude people from the same 'rights' as those who are dying (Coelho et al, 2023). Similarly, Belgium's 2014 amendment extending euthanasia to minors represents systematic removal of age-based protections through autonomy arguments. As Raus (2016, p 305) discusses, this amendment makes euthanasia legally possible for all minors judged to possess 'capacity of discernment' regardless of biological age, provided they meet other criteria. Yet the law leaves key terms like 'capacity of discernment' undefined, creating what critics identify as dangerous ambiguity in implementation.

A second mechanism operates through economic prioritisation that systematically withdraws (or limits) support for alternatives to death. Scobie et al (2025) document that in the UK, less than half of hospice funding

(44% in 2022) comes from public sources, with the remainder dependent on charitable fundraising. Yet implementing assisted dying requires – and presumably is set to receive in the UK – substantial investment in new infrastructure, including regulation and oversight bodies, data systems, specialist training and pharmacy protocols. This contrast reveals deliberate policy choices – governments find resources to create comprehensive pathways to death while leaving palliative care chronically underfunded and dependent on charity. When states systematically underinvest in alternatives to death while simultaneously investing in mechanisms to provide death, this constitutes omission by commission – formal decisions that withdraw adequate support for living while expanding access to dying.

Both mechanisms – rights expansion and economic prioritisation – systematically remove protections from vulnerable populations through different but complementary logics. Whether justified through appeals to autonomy and equality or through decisions about resource allocation priorities, the result is the same – making death more accessible while reducing safeguards for those most at risk.

Resisting ableism as a dispositif *of violence in end-of-life contexts*

Our analysis thus far has revealed assisted dying and terminalism as manifestations of ableism as violence. This raises the question: how might we resist these forces while remaining sensitive to the experiences of those who desire assisted dying?

Effective resistance, we suggest, requires approaches to end-of-life care that honour relationality and interdependence, rather than clinging to ideals, indeed *fantasies,* of independence and self-sufficiency. Dependence on others for care does not, should not, equate to loss of dignity but rather to a recognition of the conditions of life itself, as Kittay (2019) and others working in the space of feminist ethics of care have emphasised. Bishop (2016) argues, convincingly, that we urgently need social imaginaries that challenge both the 'ontotheology' (the secular religion) of neoliberalism and its obsession with 'independence' *and* the corpse-centred epistemology of modern medicine discussed earlier in this chapter. This foundational shift in perspective creates space for alternative, relational frameworks that could guide practical resistance strategies.

Maung's (2023) externalist analysis of suffering provides crucial theoretical resources that align with this relational perspective, challenging the individualistic frameworks that dominate assisted dying discourses. Unlike internalist perspectives that locate suffering within the individual, externalism recognises suffering as constitutively dependent on social–environmental contexts. This framework reveals how conditions deemed 'irremediable' often reflect inadequate social responses rather than inherent features of medical conditions. As Sallnow et al (2025, p 103) observe, 'choice depends on options, and the reality for many globally is a profound absence of options'. Expanding meaningful options beyond death requires substantial investment in palliative care, disability services, mental healthcare, and social support systems.

Of course, most importantly, effective resistance to ableism as a *dispositif* of violence must centre disabled people's collective voices and experiences. When disabled people organise collectively through groups like *Not Dead Yet*, they create counter-narratives and political resistance that challenge the thanatopolitical logic of assisted dying. These collective practices represent vectors of resistance and transformation that emerge from within and against ableism as a *dispositif* of violence. As Longmore (2005) demonstrates through a series of case studies, disabled people's opposition to assisted suicide often stems not from abstract moral positions but from concrete experiences of how medical systems and social services devalue their lives.

Human rights frameworks offer crucial tools for this resistance. The CRPD establishes rights to life (Article 10), equal recognition before the law (Article 12), and access to healthcare without discrimination (Article 25) – all of which are implicated in assisted dying practices. The UN CRPD Committee has expressed concerns about assisted dying legislation in several jurisdictions, noting potential violations of disabled people's rights. Drawing upon these concerns, advocacy organisations can challenge expansive assisted dying laws through human rights mechanisms. Legal protections should include robust safeguards against coercion, requirements to exhaust all appropriate treatments and support options before considering assisted dying, and explicit prohibitions on offering assisted dying based on disability or chronic illness alone. Most importantly, they should address the socio-economic factors that constrain 'choice' for many vulnerable individuals.

Practically, this means prioritising social interventions, such as adequate housing, personal assistance services, income support, accessible healthcare, and community inclusion, before considering assisted dying. It means recognising that what presents as an individual's 'intolerable suffering' often reflects societal failure rather than inherent features of impairment or illness. In policy contexts, it means ensuring meaningful consultation with disabled people's organisations, as specified in Article 4 (3) of the CRPD, moving beyond tokenistic inclusion to substantive dialogue about how assisted dying legislation affects disabled communities. Most importantly, it means listening to disabled people's concerns about assisted dying without dismissing them as paternalistic or opposed to autonomy.

Here, however, we must acknowledge the particular challenges facing resistance to assisted dying as a manifestation of ableism as violence. Unlike other forms of ableist violence examined in this book, opposition to assisted dying confronts sophisticated mechanisms of discursive capture that render resistance itself suspect. The framing of assisted dying as 'choice' and 'autonomy' positions any opposition as interference with individual freedom, marginalising disability perspectives as a 'minority special interest' rather than expert knowledge about living with impairment. While few medical professional bodies globally actively advocate *for* assisted dying, many have moved from clear opposition towards neutrality, potentially representing a subtler form of capture where even resistance becomes moderated by the *dispositif's* constraints on legitimate discourse. This shift from active opposition to 'balanced consideration' may reflect how thoroughly the *dispositif* has normalised assisted dying as a 'legitimate' medical option requiring neutral evaluation rather than ethical opposition. Legal and procedural capture channels the remaining resistance into technical debates about safeguards rather than fundamental challenges to the underlying logic. The very effectiveness of the *dispositif* is demonstrated by how thoroughly it has constrained the terms of debate, making resistance appear unreasonable even when rooted in legitimate concerns. This suggests both the sophistication of ableism as a *dispositif* of violence and the urgent need for new strategies that can challenge its foundational assumptions rather than merely negotiating within its predetermined parameters.

Conclusion

Throughout this chapter, we have examined assisted dying and terminalism as manifestations of ableism as violence. We have deployed our violence typology to demonstrate how they operate through multiple, interconnected forms of violence to devalue and eliminate disabled and chronically ill lives. This analysis extends our examination of ableism in relation to interpersonal violence and microaggressions (Chapter 4) and confinement (Chapter 5) to perhaps its most profound manifestation – the systematic legitimisation of disabled people's deaths through medical, legal, and social arrangements.

Our analysis has revealed how assisted dying, despite its framing as offering a compassionate choice, often functions as sophisticated thanatopolitics – a governance of death that determines whose lives are worth preserving and whose can be legitimately ended. We have shown how the global expansion of assisted dying follows a consistent pattern of weakening safeguards and broadening eligibility, exposing increasingly vulnerable populations to premature death.

While respecting the diversity of perspectives within disability communities, we maintain that a disability justice approach requires addressing the social conditions that make life appear unliveable before offering death as a solution to social problems. Throughout these manifestations of ableism, from interpersonal microaggressions to institutional confinement to the legitimisation of death, we observe consistent patterns – the devaluation of disabled lives, the normalisation of harm, the construction of disability as inherently tragic or burdensome, and the presentation of violence as care, protection, or choice. Most importantly, we have highlighted how assisted dying practices respond to social, institutional, and material problems with individual, biological solutions. Rather than addressing the social structures that make disabled lives difficult, they eliminate the individuals experiencing these difficulties.

Our analysis revealed how assisted dying operates through both our violence typology and the *dispositif's* four lines. Through *acts of commission* (direct provision of death), *omission* (failure to provide alternatives), *commission by omission* (deliberate withholding of support while offering death), and *omission by commission* (systematic removal of protections), assisted dying produces measurable harm to disabled lives. These forms of violence operate through *lines of visibility* that render certain impairments as markers of 'lives not worth living'; *lines of utterance* that privilege medical discourse over disabled people's knowledge about meaningful existence; *lines of force* that enable clinical authority to propose death while withholding supports; and *lines of subjectivation* that encourage disabled people to internalise messages about being burdens, potentially leading them to view death as reasonable rather than recognising how social conditions constrain choice.

Resistance requires multifaceted approaches – externalist frameworks that address the social–environmental contexts of suffering, the centring of disabled voices and experiences in policy development, rights-based approaches that protect vulnerable populations, and relational ethics that value interdependence over individualistic autonomy.

The central insight of our analysis is that assisted dying cannot be separated from the socio-political contexts that render some lives less grievable and more disposable than others. In resisting and working toward approaches to end-of-life care that challenge ableism as a *dispositif* of violence, we affirm the fundamental principle that all lives – regardless of ability, age, prognosis, or productivity – have inherent dignity and worth. We reject the neoliberal calculation that some lives cost too much to sustain and insist instead on building societies where everyone receives the support necessary for a dignified life until its natural end.

The patterns of violence we have identified in assisted dying contexts connect directly to our final empirical analysis. In Chapter 7, we examine how the COVID-19 pandemic has functioned as a revelatory moment that has exposed and intensified all the mechanisms of ableism as a *dispositif* of violence explored throughout this book. The pandemic has revealed how quickly the devaluation of disabled lives examined here, the institutional confinements analysed in Chapter 5, and the everyday microaggressions discussed in Chapter 4 converge during a crisis to produce systematic abandonment of disabled lives on an unprecedented scale.

Cutaway 5: Thinking together – about the *Not Dead Yet* Campaign

Miro Griffiths has been involved with the Not Dead Yet UK Campaign for over 15 years, supporting the vital work of Baroness Jane Campbell and other disabled activists. While he has supported the campaign throughout this time, his public role as a spokesperson has become more prominent in recent years, as he has presented evidence to both UK and Scottish parliamentary committees regarding assisted dying legislation.

Angharad: Miro, in our last conversation, we discussed my submission to the UN about group homes. Today, I'd like to continue exploring our academic activism by focusing on your work with *Not Dead Yet UK*. You've been involved with the campaign for a long time, haven't you?

Miro: Yes, but my involvement became more visible in response to the recent legislative proposals. When Baroness Meacher's bill in the House of Lords and Liam McArthur's Assisted Dying for Terminally Ill Adults (Scotland) Bill began gaining momentum, it became increasingly important for disabled people's voices to be heard in these debates. These bills claim to offer compassionate choice, but they fundamentally misunderstand the realities of disabled people's lives and the systemic barriers we face.

Angharad: Could you expand on what you mean by 'misunderstanding realities'?

Miro: My overwhelming concern is how assisted dying coalesces with the systemic injustices faced by disabled communities. What we've identified as 'ableism as a *dispositif* of violence' systematically devalues disabled lives. I can't stress how worried I am when I have a decline in health and go into hospital. One of the first questions medical professionals ask is if I want a DNAR order, because they make assumptions about my quality of life, irrespective of my professional responsibilities and personal relationships.

Angharad: That is horrifying.

Miro: It is. If I need adjustments or dialogue with practitioners who are familiar with my needs, I'm looking at waiting 8 to 12 weeks for an appointment. Yet the same system that makes me wait months for pain management would potentially offer assisted death within weeks.

This creates what I would call a 'twin-track approach,' where for certain populations the state facilitates death, while for others it works to prevent suicide.

Angharad: I imagine this perspective hasn't always been well-received when you've presented evidence to parliamentary committees?

Miro: It's challenging. When testifying before both the UK Parliament and Scottish Parliament committees, I've emphasised how the supposedly 'strict safeguards' cannot account for the subtle coercion disabled people already experience within healthcare settings. When discussing McArthur's bill with the Scottish Parliament's Health, Social Care and Sport Committee, I highlighted how creating a network of practitioners sympathetic to assisted dying would undermine any attempts to objectively scrutinise coercion.

Angharad: One thing that struck me about your testimony is how you connect individual experiences to broader structural issues.

Miro: That's essential to understand. These issues could be resolved by focusing on how personalised medicine and support can allow people to live as their needs change over time. But instead, we're seeing what this chapter identifies as 'neoliberal thanatopolitics' – death presented not as an imposition but as a choice or right, while obscuring the structural conditions that constrain that 'choice'.

Angharad: What about the eligibility criteria in the proposed legislation? Proponents argue these provide adequate safeguards.

Miro: The criteria are incredibly weak and broad. How do you come to an objective opinion on what constitutes 'progressive', 'advanced', or 'unable to recover'? This highlights the arbitrary nature of the six-month perspective. What constitutes six months left to live, particularly when engaging with medical technologies? If I remove my ventilator, stop using my other medical devices, and discontinue therapeutic services, would that constitute having a terminal illness because my acceleration towards death becomes more evident?

Angharad: You've raised concerns about the expansion of criteria we've seen in other countries. Do you see that as inevitable if legislation passes?

Miro: Absolutely. Prominent campaigners are advocating for assisted suicide, though many wouldn't be eligible under proposed legislation. It would be naïve to assume campaigning would stop if the legislation were passed. One of my strongest messages is: Do you want a society where everyone has access to assisted suicide? That's ultimately where this leads, unless you believe in exceptionalism.

Angharad: What gives you hope in this ongoing campaign?

Miro: What gives me hope is when people truly engage with the substance of our arguments rather than dismissing us as merely opposed to choice. We're not opposed to improving end-of-life care or expanding options. We're opposed to a fundamental shift in how the state approaches vulnerability – from protection to facilitation of death. The really compassionate response isn't offering a 'quick exit' but creating a society where everyone has the support they need to live with dignity, regardless of their impairment or health condition.

You can find out more about Miro's advocacy work with Not Dead Yet UK via the following:

Evidence to UK Parliament's Public Bill Committee at: https://hansard.parliament.uk/commons/2025-01-29/debates/183b8129-4b55-45dc-a2b1-abc677a3cfc0/TerminallyIllAdults(EndOfLife)Bill(FourthSitting) [Available: 20 September 2025].

Evidence to the Scottish Parliament's Health, Social Care and Sport Committee at: https://www.parliament.scot/chamber-and-committees/official-report/search-what-was-said-in-parliament/meeting-of-parliament-21-01-2025?meeting=16218&iob=138567 [Available: 20 September 2025].

His interview on BBC Radio 4's Today Programme at: https://drive.google.com/file/d/1l1MtGfCPeorJMbQXeOlPuF07GKHDtGd–/view [Available: 20 September 2025].

His appearance on BBC Radio 4's Moral Maze: https://www.bbc.co.uk/programmes/m001vcqm [Available: 20 September 2025].

7

Failure of human services during the COVID-19 pandemic

Around the world, the COVID-19 pandemic functioned as a critical juncture that exposed underlying social inequalities and injustices in their starkest form. For disabled people, it intensified and made visible existing mechanisms of ableism as a *dispositif* of violence, revealing how quickly protective systems collapsed under pressure. This crisis brought together all manifestations previously examined in this book – microaggressions became macroaggressions, confinement logics intensified with deadly consequences for those living in institutions, and ableist or terminalist reasoning became explicit in triage protocols. It vividly displayed all four forms of violence in our typology – *commission* (direct harm), *omission* (failures to provide care), *commission by omission* (deliberate withholding of treatment by those with discretionary powers), and *omission by commission* (systematic policies legitimising blanket abandonment or other withdrawals of support or protection).

The pandemic also revealed how the *dispositif* operated through its four interconnected lines. *Lines of utterance* were particularly evident in how media and policy discourse described or implied institutional deaths as 'tragic but inevitable', naturalising structural neglect while obscuring government responsibility; how DNAR orders were reframed as 'palliative appropriateness' rather than abandonment; and how withdrawal of social care was justified by the use of terms such as 'temporary safety suspensions' – framing systematic abandonment as protective while ignoring risks of neglect, isolation, and carer burnout. *Lines of visibility* rendered disabled people hypervisible as 'vulnerable populations' while making their actual experiences of neglect invisible in policy responses. *Lines of force* enabled medical professionals and officials to deploy discretionary authority in rationing care while claiming resource constraints, sometimes supported by legal frameworks (see, for example, in the UK, the Care Act 'easements'). *Lines of subjectivation* created conditions where disabled people were constantly exposed to messaging about their expendability and burden on healthcare systems.

What happened to disabled people during the intense crisis period of COVID-19 was not an unfortunate side effect of an emergency but rather the acceleration of ableist systems and practices that normally operate more slowly and less visibly. What happened was a textbook example of the 'slow/fast violence' complex, as described by Christian and Dowler (2019). This allowed the deaths and suffering of disabled people during the pandemic to be framed as unfortunate collateral damage (Abrams and Abbott, 2020).

As in previous chapters, we draw upon evidence from across the world, from both Majority and Minority worlds, to demonstrate that the pandemic created a crisis for disabled people *globally*. The violence of ableism during the intense crisis period of COVID-19 transcended national borders, political systems, and economic circumstances – though it manifested in contextually specific ways. As in previous chapters, we will, however, focus particular attention on the UK to examine how these global patterns played out in the context we know most intimately. The personal and the political intertwine throughout our examination. In the cutaway for this chapter, Miro reflects upon his own lived experiences during the pandemic, providing a first-person perspective that complements our broader sociological analysis.

A global catastrophe: bearing witness

Speaking at the launch of the Policy Brief on Persons with Disabilities and COVID-19 in May 2020, UN Secretary-General António Guterres warned:

> Even under normal circumstances, persons with disabilities are less likely to access education, healthcare, and income opportunities or participate in the community. This is exacerbated for those in humanitarian and fragile contexts. People with disabilities are more likely to live in poverty, and they experience higher rates of violence, neglect and abuse. The pandemic is intensifying these inequalities – and producing new threats. (UN Press Release, 2020, n.p.)

His warning proved tragically prescient.

In the UK, data from the Office for National Statistics (2022) shows that six out of ten people who died from COVID-19 were disabled, with the risk of death being 1.3–1.6 times greater for disabled people compared to their non-disabled counterparts. A study published in the *Lancet Public Health* identified that while some risk factors related to biology (age and certain impairments), the majority stemmed from social factors, such as increased exposure through care arrangements, barriers to accessing treatment, and higher rates of poverty and deprivation (Bosworth et al, 2021). These social factors reflect the operation of ableism as violence through its material, institutional, and socioeconomic dimensions.

Looking beyond the UK, Kubenz and Kiwan's (2021) review of the situation in low- and middle-income countries revealed a sharp increase in poverty, especially food poverty, among disabled people during the pandemic, with many perceiving hunger to be a bigger threat than the virus itself. Social assistance was difficult to access and frequently excluded disabled people.

The absence of formal social care placed immense pressure on informal networks, which often broke down during lockdowns, resulting in isolation, neglect, and sometimes death.

The shadow of eugenics hung over many countries' responses. In Italy, guidance from the College of Anaesthesia, Analgesia, Resuscitation and Intensive Care suggested withdrawing support based on 'presence of comorbidities' and prioritising those requiring fewer 'resource-consuming' interventions (SIAARTI, 2020, n.p.). This echoes the ableist and terminalist reasoning we examined in Chapter 6, now expanded through systematic triage protocols. It reminds us of the category of the 'useless eaters' (*Unnütze Esser*) used by the Nazi regime of 1930s Germany to 'justify' the mass killing of disabled people (Mostert, 2002). Analysing these guidelines, Montanari Vergallo et al (2021) contrasted utilitarian and deontological approaches to triage during the pandemic, arguing that the quality-of-life metrics used in such protocols unjustly privileged younger, able-bodied individuals while marginalising elderly and disabled people. 'Cutting off' entire sections of the community was tantamount to 'eugenic selection', they argued, and a 'blatant violation of common sense, medical ethics, and the fundamental principles of the rule of law, as well as numerous international provisions that directly or indirectly prohibit the use of eugenic practices' (Montanari Vergallo et al, 2021, p 6).

Media reports during the pandemic highlighted how the UK's Clinical Frailty Score had become a 'coronavirus scoring system' categorising people with learning disabilities as 'frail' even when they were healthy (Boyd, 2020). The charity Turning Point documented cases such as that of a man in his fifties with sight loss who was discharged from hospital with a DNAR order, citing his 'blindness and severe learning disabilities' as justification (Lintern, 2020, n.p.). During the pandemic, 'micro-invalidation' became 'macro-invalidation' – enacted at a systemic, not only an interpersonal level.

These patterns of deprioritisation and abandonment manifested in countless tragedies worldwide. The pandemic revealed not merely isolated incidents of neglect but systemic failures rooted in ableist structures that have long positioned disabled lives as expendable. To bear witness to this reality, we offer two illustrative cases that embody the broader patterns of structural violence experienced by disabled people during this global crisis.

In Sweden, care home nurse Latifa Löfvenberg reported to the BBC News that staff were instructed not to send residents to hospitals, regardless of their condition – even those with potentially many years left to live. She recounted, 'They told us that we shouldn't send anyone to the hospital, even if they may be 65 and have many years to live. We were told not to send them in' (quoted on BBC News, 2020, n.p.).

This approach contributed to a significant number of COVID-19 deaths among care home residents. Prime Minister Stefan Löfven later acknowledged the shortcomings in protecting the elderly, stating, 'We have not protected the most vulnerable, the most elderly, despite our best intentions' (BBC News, 2020, n.p.).

In China, Yan Cheng, a 17-year-old man who had cerebral palsy, died alone after his father and brother were forcibly quarantined. Despite his father's desperate public plea on the social media platform Weibo, it is reported that local officials only arranged for a meal to be sent to Yan twice in six days. Members of the wider community also failed to support Yan. Following his death, officials were removed from office, but a government spokesperson defensively claimed, '(i)t is definitely not true that nobody took care of him', while acknowledging that they had not 'cared for him dutifully' – exemplifying how systems can fail to take responsibility for the abandonment of disabled people at times of crisis (Shelton and Yang, 2020, n.p.).

Far from representing exceptional circumstances, these examples reveal the logical endpoint of societies that systematically devalue disabled lives. The contrast between deontological ethics, which would insist on the inherent value and dignity of all persons regardless of ability status, and the utilitarian calculations that underpinned many pandemic responses is stark. These responses did not emerge from nowhere but represent the acceleration and intensification of pre-existing ableist logics that permeate our social, medical, and political institutions.

The UK context

In the UK, the *Covid-19 Inquiry* has provided a formal space for bearing witness to the disproportionate impact of the pandemic on disabled people. Through witness statements and expert evidence, the inquiry has documented systematic failures across healthcare, social care, and public health communication – revealing not isolated incidents but patterns of violence against disabled people.

The testimony of Stringer (2023, p 7), representing the Disability Charities Consortium, to the inquiry, highlighted that '30,296 of 50,888 COVID deaths in early 2020 were of Disabled people' (figures from the Office for National Statistics). This means that six in ten deaths were of disabled people, despite them accounting for only 22% of the UK population. People with learning disabilities were particularly endangered – being six times more likely to die during the first wave, with this risk rising to 30 times higher for those aged 18 to 34. This shocking disparity cannot be explained by biology alone; rather, it reflects the operation of ableism as violence through its institutional and policy dimensions.

Some of the most disturbing evidence presented to the inquiry concerned the inappropriate application of DNAR orders to disabled people, especially, but not only, people with learning disabilities. The testimony of O'Sullivan (2024), representing The Royal Mencap Society before the inquiry, is particularly revealing in this regard. She describes doctors raising the issue of withholding resuscitation with family members who 'said they would like time to think about it, and then doctors applied a DNAR notice regardless' (O'Sullivan, 2024, p 15).

These inquiry testimonies are supported by broader research into the pandemic's impact. Warner (2023) found that during the pandemic, DNAR orders were applied to disabled people in ways that violated both legal precedent and ethical principles, representing a systematic violation of established medical duties to consult patients and families. Such practices contravened established case law. In *Tracey, R (on the Application of) v Cambridge University Hospitals NHS Foundation Trust & Ors* [2014], the Court of Appeal established that Article 8 of the Human Rights Act 1998 requires that DNAR decisions be made by consulting the patient/their family. This principle was further substantiated in *Winspear v City Hospitals Sunderland NHS Foundation Trust* [2015], where the imposition of a DNAR order on a 28-year-old man with cerebral palsy without his family's knowledge was found to be a clear violation of his Article 8 rights.

Beyond the inquiry proceedings, further evidence of institutional discrimination emerged. The Care Quality Commission (CQC, 2020) found that DNAR orders were being applied to groups rather than individuals. This included a GP sending DNAR letters to care homes asking them to put blanket orders in place. The CQC found that 3.8% of DNAR decisions put in place since 17 March 2020 had not been considered as part of a personalised care plan. In its public survey, 48% of individuals with a DNAR decision believed that they had encountered unfair or discriminatory treatment during the decision-making process'.

Inclusion London's (2020, p 16) research captured the emotional toll of such discrimination, quoting a member of their organisation as stating, 'I feel trapped and controlled and claustrophobic (…) too scared to leave the house because (…) doctors will leave me to die'.

This statement exemplifies the terror experienced by many disabled people when they realised that their lives had been officially deemed less valuable by the very systems meant to provide protection.

Returning to the formal inquiry evidence, the *Expert Report on Disability and Structural Inequalities for the UK Covid-19 Inquiry*, authored by Disability Studies researchers Watson and Shakespeare (2023), concluded that disabled people faced an elevated risk of harm from COVID-19, due in part to biological vulnerabilities but also to structural inequalities (poverty, housing, employment) and dependence on weakened health and social care systems. The *Module 1 Report of the UK Covid-19 Inquiry* (2024, n.p.) provided the salutary conclusion that 'emergency planning generally failed to account sufficiently for pre-existing health and societal inequalities'. As the Rt Hon. the Baroness Hallett DBE states in her introduction to the report: 'There must be radical reform. Never again can a disease be allowed to lead to so many deaths and so much suffering' (UK Covid-19 Inquiry, 2024, n.p.).

Institutions as death traps: confinement's deadly logic

Zooming out again from the UK, nowhere was ableism as a *dispositif* of violence more starkly revealed than in congregate settings – institutions, group homes, psychiatric facilities, and care homes. Around the world, these spaces, which we examined in Chapter 5 as sites of confinement and carceral logic, became death traps during the pandemic. The 'warehousing' of disabled bodies created the perfect conditions for viral spread, while the devaluation of disabled lives ensured that these populations would be the last to receive protective measures and the first to face abandonment.

In April 2020, the Office of the United Nations High Commissioner for Human Rights (2020) reported that preliminary studies suggested that deaths in care homes represented 42–57% of all COVID-19 deaths in many countries. This staggering figure represents the predictable outcome of systems that segregate disabled people in ways that make them uniquely vulnerable to infectious disease. Institutional residents already faced greater risks of human rights violations before the pandemic, but during the crisis, they faced heightened risks due to the impossibility of physical distancing, a lack of protective equipment, and, in some cases, abandonment by staff (Brennan et al, 2020). Further, these outcomes reflect the systematic redefinition of care duties during the crisis – transforming professional obligations to protect all residents equally into discretionary calculations about whose lives warranted scarce resources.

In the US, the National Council on Disability (2021) reported that by March 2021, 181,000 disabled people living in long-term care facilities had died from COVID-19. The European Network for Independent Living documented how, in Romania, disabled people infected with the virus were refused access to local healthcare services. Those who tested positive were 'quarantined' in separate buildings within institutions, while infected staff were hospitalised to receive immediate healthcare (Hadad et al, 2020). This disparity in treatment starkly reveals how ableism operates through both institutional arrangements and clinical decision-making.

These patterns of institutional death evidence the operation of what Ben-Moshe (2020) terms 'carceral ableism' – the intersection of disability oppression and incarceration that we explored in Chapter 5. The pandemic exposed how institutions function not as therapeutic environments but as spaces to locate and dispose of those deemed surplus to social requirements (Bauman, 2004).

Community abandonment: the collapse of support systems

Ableism as a *dispositif* of violence also operated with devastating efficiency in community contexts. The pandemic exposed the fragility of support networks and the conditional nature of societal commitments to disabled people's wellbeing. This can be seen in the tragic case of Yan Cheng – abandoned not just by local authorities, but also by his community.

Community-based support services failed disabled people during the pandemic in profound ways. Around the world, the fragility of many disabled people's support networks and their heightened risk of isolation became apparent. Personal assistance processes and mechanisms broke down as critical workers struggled to carry out their duties (International Disability Alliance, 2020). In an article for *Euronews* (Parrock, 2020, n.p.), César Giménez, a disability rights campaigner in Spain, expressed fears for his independence and dignity: 'If my personal assistant got sick, they, my parents, wouldn't be able to put me in the shower or do things for me to be able to take care of my personal hygiene'.

Alice Jorge, an activist in Belgium, spoke about having to choose between allowing infected nursing staff to visit or placing all responsibility on her sister. In both cases, the burden of navigating complex risks was placed on disabled individuals and their families rather than being addressed through systematic or indeed community (voluntary) support.

The title of Inclusion London's (2020) report, *Abandoned, forgotten and ignored*, captures disabled people's experiences during the first wave of the UK's pandemic perfectly. The report documents the exclusion of many disabled people from priority shopping lists, their struggles to access medication deliveries, and their lack of essential support. The report quotes a disabled person as follows: 'No one contacted me from social services to see if I was coping' (Inclusion London, 2020, p 19) – a stark illustration of institutional abandonment.

Goodley et al (2023) explored the affective impacts of the pandemic on disabled people through their analysis of global blog posts, where they identified heightened feelings of fragility (intensified feelings of disposability through triage frameworks and social Darwinism) and anxiety (amplified by lockdowns and loss of services). The profound impact of these experiences is captured in one disabled blogger's words: 'I am a disabled woman in a body that is labelled as weak and unworthy – disposable' (Haraldsdóttir, cited in Goodley et al, 2023, p 1195).

What is clear from all the evidence and research we have considered, is that what happened during the pandemic was not simply a failure of individual services, but a strategic and systematic abandonment of disabled people by societies and their governments. This represents not an unfortunate side effect of a crisis but the operation of ableism as a *dispositif* of violence through its institutional and systemic dimensions.

The pandemic as a revelation

The COVID-19 pandemic functioned as a 'revelatory moment' – exposing social dynamics and power relations typically obscured (for many) during ordinary times. Its significance lay not in creating new forms of discrimination, but in laying bare the ableism as a *dispositif* of violence, with unmistakable clarity.

During the pandemic, disabled people experienced a troubling paradox – simultaneously hypervisible as a 'vulnerable group' requiring protection, yet seemingly invisible in the implementation of emergency support measures. Politicians invoked 'protecting the vulnerable' to justify restrictions on the public, but failed to *actually* protect those who were truly most vulnerable.

The invisibility extended to statistical accounting – many countries failed to record disability status in COVID-19 data until disabled people's organisations protested this erasure. Meanwhile, people with learning disabilities in residential care, those with psychosocial disabilities residing in psychiatric institutions, and autistic people with high support needs vanished from public view as family visits ceased and monitoring mechanisms suspended operations.

Medical and technocratic language dominated pandemic discourse, while disabled people's experiential knowledge was systematically devalued. Triage protocols, drafted predominantly by non-disabled medical professionals, employed supposedly objective measures of 'quality of life' and 'resource consumption' that encoded ableist assumptions. When disabled activists challenged these protocols, their concerns were dismissed as 'emotional' rather than substantive – revealing how ableist discourse positions medical expertise as rational while rendering disabled people's knowledge subjective.

The necropolitics of the pandemic response

The pandemic response further exposed the necropolitical dimensions of ableism, operating as a *dispositif* of violence – marking the threshold where biopolitics (the governance of life) gave way to necropolitics (the governance of death). Drawing on Mbembe's (2003) concept, we can understand how the pandemic made visible the sovereign power to determine who may live and who must die. This necropolitical dimension connects directly to our analysis of assisted dying and terminalism in Chapter 6, where we identified how medical systems increasingly position death as an acceptable 'solution' to impairment and disability. The pandemic merely accelerated this logic, transforming what normally proceeds through individual medical decisions into systematic policy frameworks.

During the pandemic, we witnessed the operation of 'social death' on an unprecedented scale. No longer confined to individual clinical judgements about specific patients, the process of social death expanded to encompass entire categories of people deemed less valuable. The bureaucratic rationality documented by Timmermans and Sudnow (1998) in resuscitation decisions – where staff rationed their efforts based on hierarchies of lives they considered worth saving – became explicit in pandemic triage protocols and resource allocation frameworks.

In multiple jurisdictions, governments implemented policies that explicitly or implicitly designated certain populations – predominantly disabled and elderly people (many of whom were also disabled) – as *sacrificable*. These decisions were not framed as abandonment but as rational resource allocation. Cost–benefit analyses, quality–adjusted life year calculations, and triage protocols translated complex value judgements about human worth into seemingly objective metrics.

The pandemic response: working through the typology of violence

As stated at the chapter's opening, the COVID-19 pandemic provided a stark demonstration of how ableism as a *dispositif* of violence operates through all four forms in our typology, revealing mechanisms that typically remain obscured within routine healthcare and social care practices. Each form manifested with particular intensity during the crisis – their interconnected operations exposed the systematic nature of harm inflicted upon disabled people when protective systems came under pressure.

Acts of commission operated through direct harmful interventions against disabled people's bodies and lives. DNAR orders were inappropriately applied without consultation, often using assessment tools that categorised disabled people as unsuitable for treatment even when they were otherwise healthy. Medical professionals imposed life-limiting decisions based on assumptions about quality of life rather than clinical necessity. Direct abandonment also constituted commission, as disabled people were left without essential support despite family pleas and available resources to provide care.

Acts of omission manifested through systematic failures to provide essential care, protection, and support that disabled people required for survival. Healthcare systems failed to develop inclusive emergency planning despite knowing disabled people's heightened vulnerabilities. Care institutions received inadequate resources and protection. Essential support services were withdrawn without alternative provision, leaving disabled people to navigate impossible circumstances alone. These failures to act produced devastating consequences, including preventable deaths from inadequate supervision and care.

Commission by omission operated through deliberate decisions not to act, despite awareness of need and capacity to intervene. Medical professionals exercised discretionary authority to deny treatment based on quality-of-life assessments that encoded ableist assumptions about whose lives warranted saving. Triage protocols enabled the systematic deprioritisation of disabled people through seemingly neutral clinical frameworks. Officials chose not to act on available evidence of harm and neglect, using professional discretion to avoid fulfilling duties of protection and care.

Omission by commission functioned through systematic policy decisions that formally withdrew protections from disabled people under emergency justifications. Legislative frameworks enabled the reduction of statutory duties to provide social care and support. Changes to eligibility criteria for life-saving interventions effectively expanded the category of those deemed ineligible, encompassing disabled people who had previously been protected from such exclusion. Resource allocation systems were restructured to systematically disadvantage disabled people in accessing essential services. These policy changes transformed fundamental rights into conditional privileges that could be withdrawn through administrative decisions.

The pandemic response: working through the lines

Further, the pandemic exposed with unprecedented clarity how ableism as a *dispositif* of violence operates through interconnected lines that determine what can be seen, said, and done in relation to disabled people. Crisis conditions intensified these operations; the *dispositif's* strategic function became visible as protective rhetoric gave way to systematic abandonment.

Lines of visibility operated through a paradox that rendered disabled people simultaneously hypervisible and invisible within pandemic responses. Disabled people became hypervisible as 'vulnerable populations' requiring protection; this visibility justified restrictions on their movement and autonomy, while policies systematically failed to provide *actual* protection. Care homes were visible as sites of tragedy but invisible as sites of preventable neglect. Disabled people's deaths appeared in statistics, yet their experiences of abandonment remained unseen by policy makers. The visibility of disabled people as burdens on healthcare systems contrasted sharply with the invisibility of their expertise; their voices disappeared (*if they have ever been present*) from emergency planning and decision-making processes.

Lines of utterance functioned through a systematic manipulation of language that concealed violence while legitimising harm. DNAR orders became 'palliative appropriateness', transforming abandonment into therapeutic intervention. Media discourse described or implied that institutional deaths were 'tragic but inevitable', naturalising structural neglect as an unfortunate consequence of vulnerability rather than policy failure. The withdrawal of social care was rearticulated in terms of 'temporary safety suspensions', framing systematic abandonment as a protective measure.

Clinical language normalised discriminatory resource allocation through euphemisms like 'difficult decisions' and 'unprecedented circumstances', providing cover for systematic deprioritisation of disabled lives.

Lines of force manifested through power relations that enabled professionals and officials to exercise discretionary authority over disabled people's lives and deaths. Medical professionals deployed clinical authority to deny treatment and impose DNAR orders without consultation. Emergency legislation created new zones of professional discretion while suspending normal oversight mechanisms. Triage protocols enabled systematic discrimination under the guise of clinical necessity. These power relations were strategic, enabling rapid deployment of discriminatory practices while maintaining professional legitimacy.

Lines of subjectivation created conditions where disabled people faced constant messaging about their expendability and reduced claim to social resources during crises. The emphasis on protecting 'vulnerable' populations positioned disabled people as objects requiring management rather than subjects with rights. Triage frameworks communicated clear messages about whose lives were deemed worth saving. The withdrawal of services, accompanied by messaging about temporary necessity, suggested disabled people's needs were discretionary rather than essential. While time will tell how these messages have 'nurtured' internalised ableism, the conditions for such internalisation were systematically created through repeated communications about disabled people's reduced value within social systems under pressure.

Resistance within crisis: disability justice and mutual aid

While it is essential to bear witness to these catastrophic failures if we are to understand the full extent of the violence against disabled people during the pandemic, it would be a grave disservice to disabled communities to portray them solely as victims without agency or *collective* resilience. It is important to acknowledge the forms of resistance that emerged. Throughout the pandemic, disabled people developed sophisticated strategies to counter their abandonment and assert their right to exist. These acts of resistance transcended opposition to specific policies, challenging the foundational logics of ableism and disrupting the established lines that we have described within this book – *of visibility, utterance, force* and *subjectivation*.

Perhaps the most significant form of resistance was the rapid development of disability-led mutual aid networks (see Goodley et al, 2023). As Piepzna-Samarasinha (2021, n.p.) articulates, these networks drew on long-established survival strategies: 'We were sick, crazy people who were determined to stay alive'. Unlike mainstream mutual aid, disabled mutual aid operated with greater attention to accessibility, practical support, and relational trust, distributing essential supplies, coordinating remote support, sharing crucial information, and providing social connection during isolation.

Goodley et al (2023) documented how disabled people created psychopolitical spaces of affective support through digital self-advocacy, peer-led networks, and critical intervention. Similarly, Inclusion London (2020) highlighted peer networks, legal challenges, and demands for inclusion in decision-making. Epistemic resistance also emerged through alternative knowledge production. Civil society led initiatives such as the *COVID-19 Disability Rights Monitor* (https://www.covid-drm.org/) collected evidence and testimonies globally, creating an alternative archive of experiences systematically excluded from official accounts.

Legal resistance played a crucial role in challenging the pandemic's necropolitical dimensions. As Kavanagh et al (2021, p 5) noted, lobbying from advocates and academics in Australia resulted in more responsive policies, while in England, 'a high-profile campaign and legal action overturned aspects of [frailty index] guidelines'. These legal challenges represent not merely technical disputes but fundamental contestations of the necropolitical logics that position disabled lives as expendable during crisis.

In the US, the Disability Rights Education and Defense Fund filed an amicus brief (The Arc et al, 2025) arguing that ableist value judgements shaped the denial of life-sustaining treatment to Michael Hickson (see Chapter 2). While the case remains unresolved at time of writing, the brief systematically exposes how quality-of-life assessments encode discriminatory assumptions about disabled lives, potentially creating precedent for recognising such assessments as violations of civil rights protections.

These forms of resistance highlight what Foucault termed the 'strategic reversibility' of power relations within a *dispositif*. The conditions for new forms of solidarity, consciousness, and political and legal action were found within the *dispositif* itself and allowed, at least to some degree and in some spaces, for subversion and 'lines of flight'.

Conclusion: revelation *and* possibility

Throughout this chapter, we have examined how the COVID-19 pandemic functioned as a revelatory moment for understanding ableism as a *dispositif* of violence. The pandemic did not create new forms of ableism but intensified and exposed existing mechanisms through which disabled lives are devalued, controlled, and, in some cases, eliminated. By tracing how types of violence and *lines of visibility, utterance, force*, and *subjectivation* operated during this period, we have exposed the very ontology of ableism as a *dispositif* of violence – beyond individual prejudice or isolated discrimination.

What the pandemic revealed most clearly is the conditional nature of rights and protections for disabled people. When systems came under pressure, commitments to equality and inclusion quickly gave way to calculations of worth and utility. The interpersonal violence and microaggressions explored in Chapter 4 became macroaggressions during the crisis. The confinement logics examined in Chapter 5 intensified with deadly consequences. The ableist and terminalist reasoning analysed in Chapter 6 became explicit in resource allocation and triage decisions. These connections reveal how the various manifestations of ableism as a *dispositif* of violence function as part of a coherent system that produces disability as a site of disposability.

The pandemic accelerated and made visible the process of social death – the determination that certain lives are not worth living *long before* biological death occurs. During the crisis, we witnessed how this process expanded from individual clinical judgements to encompass entire categories of people through blanket resource allocation frameworks, triage protocols, and institutional practices. This systematic application of social death reveals the ultimate operation of ableism as a *dispositif* of violence – the production of hierarchies of human value that determine whose lives will be protected and whose may be sacrificed.

Yet the pandemic also revealed possibilities for resistance and transformation. The very visibility of ableism as violence during this period, created openings for challenge and change. Disabled people's collective organising, epistemic resistance, and mutual aid practices demonstrated that alternative ways of valuing lives and organising care remain possible, even during crises. These practices offer glimpses of what a post-ableist society might look like – one founded not on hierarchies of worth but on recognition of *shared vulnerability, interdependence, and relationality* (Beckett, 2006).

As we move forward from the pandemic, the crucial question becomes whether societies will learn from this revelation or engage in strategic forgetting. Will the exposed operations of ableism as a *dispositif* of violence lead to its transformation, or will lines of utterance maintain disabled deaths as 'inevitable' or 'acceptable' losses? The patterns revealed during the acute crisis persist through policy shifts. In the UK, for example, the progressive narrowing of COVID-19 vaccination eligibility has, by autumn 2025, excluded many disabled people previously deemed 'clinically extremely vulnerable' (UKHSA, 2025). Meanwhile, long COVID continues to create new populations of disabled people experiencing familiar forms of medical dismissal and abandonment – suggesting that strategic forgetting may already be underway. The answer lies not in technical improvements to emergency planning but in fundamental reconsiderations of whose lives we value and how we understand our obligations to one another.

In our final chapter, we will explore what it might mean to move beyond critique toward the dismantling of ableism as a *dispositif* of violence – to imagine and build worlds where the forms of violence we have analysed no longer structure disabled people's experiences. The pandemic, despite its immense tragedy, may yet serve as a catalyst for transformation if we refuse to forget what it has revealed about ableism and violence, and the possibility of alternative ways of doing and being.

Cutaway 6: Thinking together – living through the pandemic

Angharad: Miro, throughout this chapter, we've examined how the pandemic revealed ableism as a *dispositif* of violence through systemic failures globally. I wonder if you could share some of your personal experiences during this period. Maybe the place to begin is your life *before* COVID-19 – what was it like?

Miro: Before the pandemic, I would describe my life as full and active. Despite what medical practitioners have labelled as my 'severe' and 'life-limiting' impairment, I was thriving. I rely on a combination of human support, assistive technologies, therapies and medication to live – and by live, I mean survive and flourish – but precisely because of this wonderful assemblage, my impairment was not life-limiting at all.

Angharad: So, you had established a support system that enabled you to live fully?

Miro: Absolutely. I was very busy! I'd just started my Leverhulme Fellowship, had a great social life, enjoyed holidays with my partner, went to football matches, frequented delicatessens to sample cheeses and threw parties!

Angharad: You throw excellent parties!

Miro: I do! For me, a full life isn't just about longevity but *quality* of life, and thanks to the different types of support I had, I was living the way I wanted.

Angharad: How did that change when the pandemic began?

Miro: I was anxious from the start. I didn't need that letter from the NHS confirming I was 'clinically extremely vulnerable' – I already knew that. I was certain my support mechanisms would fail because they were already precarious. I feared I'd be denied access to medical interventions.

Angharad: And were those fears realised?

Miro: Unfortunately, yes. For many months, I was without any of my seven personal assistants. They were becoming unwell, caring for their own families, or working across multiple households with a high risk of transmission. We received no additional funding for PPE for months, and when we finally could access tests, we had no backup funding if staff tested positive.

Angharad: How did you manage during that time?

Miro: My partner and I had been living intermittently with my father. The three of us went into lockdown together. My partner took lengthy unpaid leave and suspended her doctoral research. For over a year, none of us left our property. My dad wanted to help, but he'd had two heart attacks in recent years. In the end, my partner undertook about 90 percent of the work, which was absolutely exhausting for her.

Angharad: That sounds incredibly difficult. Do you remember how I used to call you three 'The Terrific Trio'? Behind those light-hearted check-ins was genuine anxiety for you all.

Miro: It *was* difficult. With just the three of us, I struggled with not wanting to ask too much. I tried to minimise my requests because I was conscious of the impact on their wellbeing. What was particularly distressing was how my situation was never acknowledged by my local authority. That for lengthy periods, two people were providing 24-hour care to me – work that was usually shared between seven staff.

Angharad: What about your interactions with healthcare professionals?

Miro: Contact with my regular medical professionals continued remotely. Those familiar with my needs emphasised the importance of shielding. But they also told me, honestly, and *in secret*, that they couldn't guarantee my access to medical services if I were hospitalised. It was clear somebody with my condition would not be prioritised for treatment. This was devastating news and felt like a huge threat to my life.

Angharad: And then, of course, it happened – despite all efforts to shield – you caught COVID-19.

Miro: It was terrifying. Fortunately, by then I'd had several vaccinations. But it remains one of the worst acute illnesses I've ever experienced. My temperature couldn't be regulated. I struggled to take enough breaths every minute and had uncontrollable pain. The assistive technologies I'd typically use once daily for breathing and coughing were constantly in use.

I was eligible for fast-track antiviral medication, but after notifying the local health service, it took over six days for them to contact me. By then, they said it was too late for antivirals to be effective. The clinician concluded with these words, 'Regrettably, you are on your own – we do not have any additional interventions available'.

Angharad: That phrase, 'you are on your own', seems to encapsulate much of what we've documented in this chapter.

Miro: Exactly. I felt abandoned by the state and health and social care services. The messages from government departments emphasised individual responsibility. I had to register for support rather than it being automatic. I was encouraged to contact charities and volunteer associations, which made support feel like a gift rather than the fulfilment of a basic human right. I was not only frightened but *very angry*.

Angharad: Looking back now, what conclusions do you draw from your experiences?

Miro: I learnt that when disaster struck, disabled people and their families were abandoned in fundamental ways. Those alarmingly honest calls from my doctors saying they couldn't guarantee medical help if I were hospitalised brought home that protecting me, saving me, wasn't considered a priority. My life, and that of other disabled people, was considered less valuable.

I felt the full operation of ableism as a *dispositif* of violence during the pandemic. I was left to navigate the crisis with minimal support while watching society accept disabled deaths as inevitable. I understand painfully well how others less fortunate than me did not survive, and this leaves me with profound sadness and anger.

Angharad: I'm so very glad you survived! Your story is both a powerful testament to the failures of our systems and to the determination and resourcefulness of 'The Terrific Trio'.

Miro: Yes. In many ways I think the way my father, partner, and I survived the pandemic was our collective act of resistance. That said, I know that my position is of someone relatively privileged – having my own adapted home and vital assistive technologies, not being alone, having sufficient funds to source my own PPE, and being digitally connected – offered me a somewhat greater chance of surviving than many other disabled people.

Angharad: Your experience shines a light, so clearly, on how the pandemic didn't so much *create* new forms of violence but rather it intensified *existing* mechanisms of ableism. It made visible what had been there all along.

Miro: That's precisely it. The pandemic pulled back the curtain on what many disabled people already knew – that our value is conditional, our care is precarious, and our lives are considered more expendable. What's crucial now is that we don't allow that knowledge to be buried again as society moves on.

8

Not a conclusion

To conclude a book on ableism as a *dispositif* of violence would suggest a neatness, a closure, that would contradict both our theoretical framework and our ethical commitments. Ableism as a *dispositif* of violence operates not as a static system but as a dynamic network that continuously reconfigures in response to resistance and changing conditions. In response to such a dynamic network, our analysis must remain ongoing, adaptive, and open-ended.

This, then, is *not* a conclusion, but a pause – a moment to reflect on the journey we have taken together and to consider what might lie ahead.

Moving beyond critique requires understanding how transformative practices might disrupt the mechanisms of ableism as a *dispositif* of violence that we have traced throughout this book. While systematic analysis of how such alternatives operate through our theoretical frameworks represents crucial future work – which we intend to undertake – existing practices of resistance point toward broader possibilities for transformation.

Our reconceptualisation of ableism as a *dispositif* of violence and our typology of acts of violence have allowed us to articulate and understand how violence manifests across seemingly disparate domains and practices. Through examining how the *dispositif* operates via its four interconnected lines – *lines of visibility, utterance, force, and subjectivation* – and alongside our four-part violence typology, we have revealed the systematic nature of harm inflicted upon disabled people. From hate crimes to microaggressions, from confinement to assisted dying, from interpersonal violence to pandemic response – we have traced the operation of a coherent system that renders disabled lives as less valuable and thus expendable. Our typology's focus on duty manipulation reveals how different forms of violence operate through distinct mechanisms of power, requiring correspondingly different analytical and political responses.

By grounding our analysis in embodied harm, we have emphasised that even subtle forms of violence produce measurable consequences for disabled people's bodies and minds. The different forms of violence inflicted on disabled people do not operate in isolation but simultaneously reinforce each other, as we saw vividly illustrated during the pandemic.

Implications for knowledge and practice

For scholars and researchers, we propose that our framework offers analytical precision through both the violence typology and the *dispositif* conceptualisation. The four-part typology identifies forms of violence and harm often rendered invisible within traditional paradigms. Meanwhile, our theoretical understanding of ableism as a *dispositif* of violence illuminates how these forms operate as part of a heterogeneous network of discourses, institutions, practices, and material arrangements. The four lines of the *dispositif* reveal how power operates through determining what can be seen, said, and done in relation to disabled people, while shaping how disabled people understand themselves as subjects. This dual approach opens new research directions in legal studies, institutional analysis, and examination of resistance practices.

For disability activists and advocates, our typology provides crucial language to identify and contest the full spectrum of violence against disabled people, while the *dispositif* framework connects seemingly separate struggles as manifestations of the same underlying system. Our analysis of discretionary power draws attention to key sites for intervention through the transformation of professional cultures. Simultaneously, our focus on omission by commission highlights the importance of contesting policy frameworks that withdraw protection while presenting such withdrawal as administrative necessity – revealing the strategic violence embedded in seemingly neutral governance practices.

For human rights defenders, our work helps identify and articulate rights violations through both the typology and *dispositif* analysis. The typology creates a bridge between lived experience and legal mechanisms, potentially strengthening advocacy. The *dispositif* framework exposes how human rights instruments themselves can become implicated in violence through exceptions clauses and medicalised approaches.

Moving forward together

Thankfully, while ableism as a *dispositif* of violence is powerful, it is not impenetrable or immutable. It contains contradictions and points of weakness that create openings for transformation and 'lines of flight'. Throughout our analysis, we have highlighted how disabled people and their allies resist, subvert, and reimagine – creating alternative practices and communities even within hostile systems through independent living movements, mutual aid networks, and disability justice organising. The protests, advocacy, legal challenges, and cultural interventions that we have examined demonstrate that even as the *dispositif* adapts, so too do strategies for challenging it. As Griffiths (2023) suggests, disability activism increasingly generates heterotopian counter-sites – spaces fostering alternative political imaginaries grounded in resistance. We need to build those sites as never before.

Having mapped the terrain of violence against disabled people, we find ourselves filled not with despair but with hope and determination.

Understanding how violence operates is not the same as accepting its necessity or inevitability. On the contrary, it is the first step toward imagining and creating something different. The framework developed here creates the foundation for future research that systematically explores how transformative practices might counter the forms of violence in our typology, while operating through different lines of the *dispositif*.

Our analysis does reveal, however, an important pattern and one we want to emphasise: resistance flourishes most visibly in domains where the *dispositif's* capture is less complete – in interpersonal interactions, community organising, and collective advocacy. Where 'lines of flight' appear more constrained – within institutional walls or at life's end – this is evidence of how the *dispositif* operates most intensively. Such differential zones of possibility reveal in the starkest manner the strategic operations of ableist violence, showing us precisely where the most urgent interventions are needed.

We hope this book will contribute to ongoing conversations and struggles. We offer it with humility about its limitations and hope for its potential to support the collective work of dismantling ableism and building more just worlds. That work continues beyond these pages – in communities and movements, in policy debates and courtrooms, in cultural productions, and in those everyday acts of resistance, and in the care we give to our families, friends, and neighbours.

We invite you to join us, not in concluding but in *continuing* – continuing to question, to challenge, to imagine, and to create better futures.

References

Abbott, D., Coleman-Fountain, E. and Humphrey, H. (2025) 'Disabled people negotiate gender, sexual identity and self-directed social care support in England: How does choice and control operate?', *Critical and Radical Social Work*, 13(1), pp 112–128.

Abrams, T. and Abbott, D. (2020) 'Disability, deadly discourse, and collectivity amid coronavirus (COVID-19)', *Scandinavian Journal of Disability Research*, 22(1), pp 168–174.

Adame, A.L. (2013) '"There needs to be a place in society for madness": The psychiatric survivor movement and new directions in mental health care', *Journal of Humanistic Psychology*, 54(4), pp 456–475.

Agamben, G. (2009) *'What Is an Apparatus?' and Other Essays*. Translated by D. Kishik and S. Pedatella. Stanford, CA: Stanford University Press.

Ahmed, S. (2004) 'Affective economies', *Social Text*, 22(2), pp 117–139.

Annamma, S.A., Connor, D.J. and Ferri, B.A. (2016) 'Touchstone text: Dis/ability critical race studies (DisCrit): Theorizing at the intersections of race and dis/ability', in Connor, D.J., Ferri, B.A. and Annamma, S.A. (eds) *DisCrit: Disability Studies and Critical Race Theory in Education* [online], New York: Teachers College Press, pp 9–32.

Annamma, S.A. (2018) *The Pedagogy of Pathologization: Dis/abled Girls of Color in the School–Prison Nexus*, New York: Routledge.

Arstein-Kerslake, A. and Flynn, E. (2016) 'The general comment on Article 12 of the Convention on the Rights of Persons with Disabilities: A roadmap for equality before the law', *The International Journal of Human Rights*, 20(4), pp 471–490.

Bauman, Z. (1997) *Postmodernity and Its Discontents*. Oxford: Polity.

Bauman, Z. (1989) *Modernity and the Holocaust*, Cambridge: Polity Press.

Bauman, Z. (2004) *Wasted Lives: Modernity and Its Outcasts*, Cambridge: Polity Press.

BBC News (2020) 'Coronavirus: What's going wrong in Sweden's care homes?', 18 May. Available at: https://www.bbc.co.uk/news/world-europe-52704836 (Accessed: 26 April 2025).

Beckett, A.E. (2006) *Citizenship and Vulnerability: Disability and Issues of Social and Political Engagement*, Basingstoke: Palgrave Macmillan.

Beckett, A.E. (2021) *Submission to the UN CRC Committee: On Group Homes as a form of Alternative Care for Children with Disabilities*, University of Leeds, Leeds.

Beckett, A.E. (2025) 'Rethinking disability law: Theoretical limitations and transformative possibilities', *Ars Vivendi Journal*, 17, pp 2–24.

Beckett, A.E. and Campbell, T. (2015) 'The social model of disability as an oppositional device', *Disability & Society*, 30(2), pp 270–283.

Ben-Moshe, L. (2011) 'The Contested meaning of 'Community' in Discourses of Deinstitutionalization and Community Living in the Field of Developmental Disability', in Carey, A.C. and Scotch, R.K. (ed) *Disability and Community (Research in Social Science and Disability, Vol. 6)*, Leeds: Emerald Group Publishing Limited, pp 241–264.

Ben-Moshe, L. (2020) *Decarcerating Disability: Deinstitutionalization and Prison Abolition*, Minneapolis: University of Minnesota Press.

Beresford, P. (2020) '"Mad", Mad Studies and advancing inclusive resistance', *Disability & Society*, 35(8), pp 1337–1342.

Beresford, P. and Rose, D. (2023) 'Decolonising global mental health: The role of Mad Studies', *Cambridge Prisms: Global Mental Health*, 10, e30, pp 1–8.

Bishop, J.P. (2016) 'From anticipatory corpse to posthuman god', *Journal of Medicine and Philosophy*, 41(6), pp 679–695.

Boler, M. (2004) *Feeling Power: Emotions and Education*, New York: Routledge.

Borg, K. (2015) 'Conducting critique: Reconsidering Foucault's engagement with the question of the subject', *Symposia Melitensia*, 11, pp 1–15.

Borg, K. (2018) 'Narrating disability, trauma and pain: The doing and undoing of the self in language', *Word and Text: A Journal of Literary Studies and Linguistics*, VIII, pp 169–186.

Borg, K. (2022) 'The time of our life is a political matter', *SHARE: Philosophy Sharing Foundation*, April, pp 18–20.

Bosworth, M.L., Ayoubkhani, D., Nafilyan, V., Foubert, J., Glickman, M., Davey, C. and Kuper, H. (2021) 'Deaths involving COVID-19 by self-reported disability status during the first two waves of the COVID-19 pandemic in England: A retrospective, population-based cohort study', *The Lancet Public Health*, 6(11), pp e817–e825.

Boyd, C. (2020) 'Fury over NHS 'coronavirus scoring system' which treats learning disability patients like a 'sub-class of the population'', *Daily Mail*, 13 April. Available at: https://www.dailymail.co.uk/news/article-8214689/Fury-NHS-coronavirus-scoring-discriminates-against-learning-disability-patient.html (Accessed: 18 April 2025).

Boyd, M. (2020) 'NHS using "coronavirus scoring system to decide which patients receive critical care"', *The Telegraph*, April 2020.

Brennan, C.S. (2020) *Disability Rights During the Pandemic: A Global Report on Findings of the COVID-19 Disability Rights Monitor*, Disability Rights Monitor. Available at: https://www.internationaldisabilityalliance.org/sites/default/files/disability_rights_during_the_pandemic_report_web_pdf_1.pdf (Accessed: 28 April 2025).

Brown, K. (2011) ''Vulnerability': Handle with care', *Ethics and Social Welfare*, 5(3), pp 313–321.

Burch, L. (2021) *Understanding Disability and Everyday Hate*, Cham, Switzerland: Palgrave Macmillan.

Burstow, B. (2015) *Psychiatry and the Business of Madness: An Ethical and Epistemological Accounting*, New York: Palgrave Macmillan.

Butler, J. (2004) *Precarious Life: The Powers of Mourning and Violence*, London: Verso.

Butler, J. (2009) *Frames of War: When Is Life Grievable?*, London: Verso.

Calabria, V. and Cullen, L. (2024) 'Deinstitutionalisation and the move to community care: Comparing the changing dimensions of mental healthcare after 1922 in the Republic of Ireland and England', *History of Psychiatry*, 35(2), pp 141–157.

Campbell, F.K. (2001) 'Inciting legal fictions: "Disability's" date with ontology and the ableist body of law', *Griffith Law Review*, 10(1), pp 43–63. Available at: https://research-repository.griffith.edu.au/server/api/core/bitstreams/bdf45182-e5b6-59f6-8285-2c44ad749a65/content (Accessed: 20 November 2025).

Campbell, F.K. (2008) 'Exploring internalized ableism using critical race theory', *Disability & Society*, 23(2), pp 151–162.

Campbell, F.K. (2009) *Contours of Ableism: The Production of Disability and Abledness*, Basingstoke: Palgrave Macmillan.

Campbell, F.K. (2015) 'Legislating disability: negative ontologies and the government of legal identities', in Tremain, S. (ed) *Foucault and the Government of Disability*, Ann Arbor, MI: University of Michigan Press, pp 108–130.

Care Quality Commission (CQC) (2020) *Review of Do Not Attempt Cardiopulmonary Resuscitation Decisions during the COVID-19 Pandemic. Interim Report*, London: CQC.

Castrodale, M.A. (2017) 'Critical disability studies and Mad Studies: Enabling new pedagogies in practice', *Canadian Journal for the Study of Adult Education*, 29(1), pp 49–66.

Cheng, M. (2023) 'In Canada, euthanasia is now a treatment for many non-terminal illnesses', *Associated Press*, 13 October. Available at: https://apnews.com/article/canada-euthanasia-deaths-doctors-nonterminal-nonfatal-cases-cd7ff24c57c15a404347df289788ef6d (Accessed: 27 April 2025).

Children's Commissioner for England (2015) *Unlocking potential: A study of the isolation of children in custody in England*, London: Office of the Children's Commissioner.

Christian, J.M. and Dowler, L. (2019) 'Slow and fast violence: A feminist critique of temporalities of violence', *ACME: An International Journal for Critical Geographies*, 18(5), pp 1064–1085.

Clare, E. (2015) *Exile and Pride: Disability, Queerness and Liberation* (2nd edn), Durham, NC: Duke University Press.

Clough, B. (2017) 'Disability and vulnerability: Challenging the capacity/incapacity binary', *Social Policy and Society*, 16(3), pp 469–481.

Clough, B. (2022) *The Spaces of Mental Capacity Law: Moving Beyond Binaries*, Abingdon, Oxon: Routledge.

Clough, B. (2025) 'Temporal disruptions in the UNCRPD: An untimely future for legal capacity?', *Human Rights Law Review*, 25(2), pp1–21.

Coelho, R., Maherl, J., Sonu Gaind, K. and Lemmens, T. (2023) 'The realities of medical assistance in dying in Canada', *Palliative and Supportive Care*, 21(5), pp 871–878.

Colleran, M. and Doherty, A. (2024) 'Examining assisted suicide and euthanasia through the lens of healthcare quality', *Irish Journal of Medical Ethics*, 193(1), pp 353–362.

Committee on the Rights of Persons with Disabilities (2014) *General Comment No. 1: Article 12 – Equal recognition before the law. CRPD/C/GC/1*, Geneva: United Nations.

Committee on the Rights of Persons with Disabilities (2017) *General comment No. 5 (2017) on living independently and being included in the community.* UN Doc CRPD/C/GC/5. Available at: https://digitallibrary.un.org/record/1311739 (Accessed: 29 April 2025).

Committee on the Rights of Persons with Disabilities (2018) *General Comment No. 6: Article 5 – Equality and non-discrimination. CRPD/C/GC/6.* Available at: https://digitallibrary.un.org/record/1626976?ln=en (Accessed: 23 April 2025).

Davies, S. (2024) *Disabled People and Health Inequality During COVID-19: Evidence from Wales*, Cardiff: Disability Wales.

Davis, L.J. (1995) *Enforcing Normalcy: Disability, Deafness, and the Body*, London: Verso.

de Finney, S., Dean, M., Loiselle, E. and Saraceno, J. (2011) 'All children are equal, but some are more equal than others: Minoritization, structural inequities, and social justice praxis in residential care', *International Journal of Child, Youth and Family Studies*, 2(3/4), pp 361–384.

Deleuze, G. (1992) 'What is a dispositif?', in Armstrong, T.J. (ed) *Michel Foucault: Philosopher*, New York: Routledge, pp 159–168.

Deleuze, G. and Guattari, F. (2004) *A Thousand Plateaus: Capitalism and Schizophrenia*, Translated by B. Massumi, London: Continuum.

de Vries, E., Leal Arenas, F.A., van der Heide, A., Gempeler, F., Murillo, R, Morales, O. et al (2021) 'Medical decisions concerning the end of life for cancer patients in three Colombian hospitals – a survey study', *BMC Palliative Care*, 20, 161.

Disability Rights International (DRI) (2013) *A Dead End for Children: Bulgaria's Group Homes*, Washington, DC: DRI.

Disability Rights International (DRI) (2022) *Left Behind in the War: Dangers Facing Children with Disabilities in Ukraine's Orphanages*, Washington, DC: DRI.

Disability Rights International (DRI) and Kenyan Association for the Intellectually Handicapped (KAIH) (2018) *Infanticide and Abuse: Killing and Confinement of Children with Disabilities in Kenya*, Washington, DC: DRI.

Disability Rights International (DRI) (2013) *The Rights of Children with Disabilities in Kenya: A Report on Human Rights Violations in Kenyan Institutions*, Washington, DC: DRI.

Disability Rights International (DRI) and Colectivo Vida Independiente (2018) *Still in Harm's Way: International Voluntourism, Segregation and Abuse of Children in Guatemala*, Washington, DC: DRI.

Ebben, H. (2019) *Representing autism as a discourse within ableist economies of doubt*, PhD thesis, Sheffield Hallam University.

Emerson, E., and Llewellyn, G. (2023) Exposure of women with and without disabilities to violence and discrimination: Evidence from cross-sectional national surveys in 29 middle- and low-income countries, *Journal of Interpersonal Violence*, 38(11–12), pp 7215–7241.

Erevelles, N. and Minear, A. (2010) 'Unspeakable offenses: Untangling race and disability in discourses of intersectionality', *Journal of Literary & Cultural Disability Studies*, 4(2), pp 127–145.

European Union Agency for Fundamental Rights (FRA) (2012) *Involuntary Placement and Involuntary Treatment of Persons with Mental Health Problems*, Luxembourg: Publications Office of the European Union.

Euser, S., Alink, L.R.A., Tharner, A., van IJzendoorn, M.H. and Bakermans-Kranenburg, M.J. (2016) 'The prevalence of child sexual abuse in out-of-home care: Increased risk for children with a mild intellectual disability', *Journal of Applied Research in Intellectual Disabilities*, 29(1), pp 83–92.

Feely, M. (2016) 'Disability studies after the ontological turn: A return to the material world and material bodies without a return to essentialism', *Disability & Society*, 31(7), pp 863–883.

Finegan, T. (2024) 'Assisted suicide and slippery slopes: Reflections on Oregon', *The New Bioethics*, 30(2), pp 89–102.

Finkelhor, D. and Asdigian, N.L. (1996) 'Risk factors for youth victimization: Beyond a lifestyles/routine activities theory approach', *Violence and Victims*, 11(1), pp 3–19.

Flynn, S. (2020) 'Theorising disability in child protection: Applying critical disability studies to the elevated risk of abuse for disabled children', *Disability & Society*, 35(6), pp 949–971.

Foucault, M. (1980) 'The Confession of the Flesh', in Gordon, C. (ed) *Power/Knowledge: Selected Interviews and Other Writings, 1972–1977*, Translated by C. Gordon, L. Marshall, J. Mepham and K. Soper, Brighton: Harvester Press, pp 194–228.

Foucault, M. (1982) 'The subject and power', *Critical Inquiry*, 8(4), pp 777–795.

Foucault, M. (1991) *Discipline and Punish: The Birth of the Prison*, Translated by A. Sheridan, London: Penguin.

Foucault, M. (1998) *The Will to Knowledge: The History of Sexuality, Volume 1*, Translated by R. Hurley, London: Penguin.

Foucault, M. (2007) *The Politics of Truth*. Edited by S. Lotringer. Translated by L. Hochroth and C. Porter. Los Angeles: Semiotext(e).

Fulone, I., Barreto, J.O.M., Barbareto-Filho, S., Bergamaschi, C. de C., Silva, M.T. and Lopes, L.C. (2021) 'Improving care for deinstitutionalised people with mental disorders: Experiences of the use of knowledge translation tools', *Frontiers in Psychiatry*, 12, p 575108.

Fylkesnes, I. (2021) 'Institutional talk and practices: A journey into small group-homes for intellectually disabled children', *Disability & Society*, 36(6), pp 999–1020.

García-Cuéllar, M.M., Pastor-Moreno, G., Ruiz-Pérez, I. and Henares-Montiel, J. (2023) 'The prevalence of intimate partner violence against women with disabilities: A systematic review of the literature', *Disability and Rehabilitation*, 45(1), pp 1–8.

Gauci, V. (2020) 'Dis/ability-producing technology assemblages and networks at the workplace: A new materialist analysis', *Disability & Society*, 36(3), pp 488–507.

Gleeson, B. (1999) *Geographies of Disability*, London: Routledge.

Goffman, E. (1968a) *Stigma: Notes on the Management of Spoiled Identity*, Harmondsworth: Penguin.

Goffman, E. (1968b) *Asylums: Essays on the Social Situation of Mental Patients and Other Inmates*, Harmondsworth: Penguin.

Goodley, D. (2014) *Dis/ability Studies: Theorising Disablism and Ableism*, London: Routledge.

Goodley, D., Lawthom, R., Liddiard, K. and Runswick-Cole, K. (2023) 'Affect, dis/ability and the pandemic', *Sociology of Health & Illness*, 45(6), pp 1187–1204.

Gurbai, S. (2020) 'Beyond the pragmatic definition? The right to non-discrimination of persons with disabilities in the context of coercive interventions', *Health and Human Rights*, 22(1), pp 279–292.

Grech, S. (2015) *Decolonising Disability: Thinking and Acting Globally*. Oxford: Routledge.

Griffiths, M. (2023) 'Declare independence. Independent living, oppositional devices, and heterotopias', *International Journal of Disability and Social Justice*. 2023. Vol. 3 (1), pp 24–41.

Grue, J. (2022) 'The death of others. On the narrative rhetoric of neoliberal thanatopolitics', *Disability Studies Quarterly*, 42(1).

Hadad, M., Meriluoto, S., Williams, F. and Kole, A. (2020) *People Living in Institutions are at Risk due to COVID-19*, Brussels: European Network on Independent Living.

Hadad, R., Priestley, M., Cabezas, M., Inselberg, S.H. and Uldry, M. (2020) *Report on the Situation of Persons with Disabilities in Institutions in Romania During COVID-19*, Brussels: European Network for Independent Living.

Hall, C., Raitakari, S. and Juhila, K. (2021) 'Deinstitutionalisation and "home turn" policies: Promoting or hampering social inclusion?', *Social Inclusion*, 9(3), pp 179–189.

Hall, E. (2019) 'A critical geography of disability hate crime', *Area*, 51(2), pp 249–256.

Hamraie, A. (2017) *Building Access: Universal Design and the Politics of Disability*, Minneapolis: University of Minnesota Press.

Hamraie, A. and Fritsch, K. (2019) 'Crip technoscience manifesto', *Catalyst: Feminism, Theory, Technoscience*, 5(1), pp 1–34.

Han, C. (2024) *Terminal bodies and medical authority: Rethinking death and diagnosis in critical care*, Thesis, Durham University.

Health Canada (2022) *Third annual report on Medical Assistance in Dying in Canada 2021*, Ottawa: Government of Canada. Available at: https://www.canada.ca/en/health-canada/services/publications/health-system-services/annual-report-medical-assistance-dying-2021.html (Accessed: 27 April 2025).

Health Canada (2024) *Fifth Annual Report on Medical Assistance in Dying in Canada, 2023*. Ottawa: Health Canada. Available at: https://www.canada.ca/en/health-canada/services/publications/health-system-services/annual-report-medical-assistance-dying-2023.html (Accessed: 2 November 2025).

Healy, J.C. (2020) 'It spreads like a creeping disease': Experiences of victims of disability hate crimes in austerity Britain', *Disability & Society*, 35(2), pp 176–200.

Helton, J.J., Gochez-Kerr, T. and Gruber, E. (2017) 'Sexual abuse of children with learning disabilities', *Child Maltreatment*, 23(2), pp 157–165.

Heyer, K. (2015) *Rights Enabled: The Disability Revolution, From the US, to Germany and Japan, to the United Nations*, Ann Arbor: University of Michigan Press.

Hollomotz, A. (2012) 'Disability and the continuum of violence', in Roulstone, A. and Mason-Bish, H. (eds) *Disability, Hate Crime and Violence*, London: Routledge, pp 52–63.

Holness, W. (2021) 'Hate crime based on disability in South Africa: Lessons for law reform', *SA Crime Quarterly*, 70, pp 2–19.

Hughes, B. (2012) 'Fear, pity and disgust: Emotions and the non-disabled imaginary', in Watson, N., Roulstone, A. and Thomas, C. (eds) *Routledge Handbook of Disability Studies*, London: Routledge, pp 67–78.

Hughes, K., Bellis, M.A., Jones, L., Wood, S., Bates, G., Eckley, L., McCoy, E., Mikton, C., Shakespeare, T. and Officer, A. (2012) 'Prevalence and risk of violence against adults with disabilities: A systematic review and meta-analysis of observational studies', *The Lancet*, 379(9826), pp 1621–1629.

Human Rights Watch (2016a) *'It is My Dream to Leave This Place': Children with Disabilities in Serbian Institutions*, New York: Human Rights Watch.

Human Rights Watch (2016b) *Witness: As If My Child Were a Burden to Me*. 8 June. Available at: https://www.hrw.org/news/2016/06/08/witness-if-my-child-were-burden-me (Accessed: 20 November 2025).

Human Rights Watch (2017) *Children with Disabilities: Deprivation of Liberty in the Name of Care and Treatment*, New York: Human Rights Watch.

Human Rights Watch (2019) *'They Don't Understand That We're Human Beings': The Abuse of Children and Adults with Disabilities in State Care in Kazakhstan*, New York: Human Rights Watch.

Human Rights Watch (2020) *Human Rights Dimensions of COVID-19 Response*, New York: Human Rights Watch.

Hurley, B. (2022) 'Paralympian claims Canada offered to euthanise her after she requested a stairlift', *The Independent*, 4 December. Available at: https://www.independent.co.uk/news/world/americas/christine-gauthier-paralympian-euthanasia-canada-b2238319.html (Accessed: 28 April 2025).

Hutcheon, E.J. and Lashewicz, B. (2020) 'Tracing and troubling continuities between ableism and colonialism in Canada', *Disability & Society*, 35(5), pp 695–714.

Inclusion London (2020) *Abandoned, Forgotten and Ignored: The Impact of COVID-19 on Disabled People*. Available at: https://www.inclusionlondon.org.uk/wp-content/uploads/2020/10/Abandoned-Forgotten-and-Ignored-Final.pdf (Accessed: 1 April 2025).

International Disability Alliance (2020) *Toward a Disability-Inclusive COVID-19 Response: 10 Recommendations*. Available at: https://www.internationaldisabilityalliance.org/sites/default/files/ida_recommendations_for_disability-inclusive_covid19_response_pl.pdf (Accessed: 28 April 2025).

Johnk, L. (2021) *Shifting roots: Reimagining the genealogical roots of disability studies and Mad studies through women of color feminisms*, PhD thesis, Oregon State University.

Kafer, A. (2013) *Feminist, Queer, Crip*, Bloomington: Indiana University Press.

Kattari, S.K. (2019) 'The development and validation of the Ableist Microaggression Scale', *Journal of Social Service Research*, 45(3), pp 400–417.

Kattari, S.K. (2020) 'Ableist microaggressions and the mental health of disabled adults', *Community Mental Health Journal*, 56(6), pp 1170–1179.

Kavanagh, A.M., Dickinson, H., Carey, G., Llewellyn, G., Emerson, E., Disney, G. and Hatton, C. (2021) 'Improving health care for disabled people in COVID-19 and beyond: Lessons from Australia and England', *Disability and Health Journal*, 14(2), 101050.

Keller, R.M. and Galgay, C.E. (2010) 'Microaggressive experiences of people with disabilities', in Sue, D.W. (ed) *Microaggressions and Marginality: Manifestation, Dynamics, and Impact*, Hoboken, NJ: Wiley, pp 241–268.

Kittay, E.F. (2019) *Love's Labor: Essays on Women, Equality, and Dependency* (2nd edn), New York: Routledge.

Knaul, F.M., Farmer, P.E., Krakauer, E.L., De Lima, L., Bhadelia, A., Jiang Kwete, X., et al (2018) 'Alleviating the access abyss in palliative care and pain relief – an imperative of universal health coverage: The Lancet Commission report', *The Lancet*, 391(10128), pp 1391–1454.

Kubenz, V. and Kiwan, D. (2021) *The Impact of the COVID-19 Pandemic on Disabled People in Low- and Middle-Income Countries: A Literature Review*, Birmingham: University of Birmingham.

Lawson, A. and Beckett, A.E. (2021) 'The social and human rights models of disability: Towards a complementarity thesis', *The International Journal of Human Rights*, 25(2), pp 348–379.

Lee, L., Kamenov, K., Fellinghauer, C., Sabariego, C., Chatterji, S. and Cieza, A. (2022) 'WHO Functioning and Disability Disaggregation (FDD11) tool: a reliable approach for disaggregating data by disability', *Archives of Public Health*, 80(1), 249. Available at: https://doi.org/10.1186/s13690-022-01001-2 (Accessed: 28 April 2025).

LeFrancois, B.A., Menzies, R. and Reaume, G. (eds) (2013) *Mad Matters: A Critical Reader in Canadian Mad Studies*, Toronto: Canadian Scholars Press.

Lemmens, T. (2023) 'When death becomes therapy: Canada's troubling normalisation of health care provider ending of life', *The American Journal of Bioethics*, 23(11), pp 79–84.

Liasidou, A. and Gregoriou, A. (2021) 'A longitudinal analysis of disability-related interpersonal violence and some implications for violence prevention work', *Journal of Interpersonal Violence*, 36(15–16), pp NP8687–NP8705.

Lintern, S. (2020) 'Coronavirus: Unlawful do not resuscitate orders imposed on people with learning disabilities', *The Independent*, 13 June. Available at: https://www.independent.co.uk/news/health/coronavirus-do-not-resuscitate-dnr-learning-disabilities-turning-point-a9561201.html (Accessed: 28 April 2025).

Longmore, P.K. (2003) *Why I Burned My Book and Other Essays on Disability*, Philadelphia, PA: Temple University Press.

Lord, J.E., Pons, W.I., Stein, M.A., Ellem, K. and Harpur, P. (2024) 'Disability hate speech and hate crimes: Assessing the role of the Convention on the Rights of Persons with Disabilities in tackling disability-based animus', in Burch, L. and Wilkin, D. (eds) *Disability Hate Crime: Perspectives for Change*, Abingdon, Oxfordshire: Routledge, pp 148–165.

Lorenz, F. (2020) 'Practicing silence about staff violence in residential care for children with disabilities', *Social Work & Society*, 18(3), pp 1–17. Available at: https://ejournals.bib.uni-wuppertal.de/index.php/sws/article/view/682/1297 (Accessed: 27 April 2025).

Macdonald, S.J., Donovan, C. and Clayton, J. (2023) 'I may be left with no choice but to end my torment: Disability and intersectionalities of hate crime', *Disability & Society*, 38(1), pp 127–147.

Macpherson, W. (1999) The Stephen Lawrence Inquiry: Report of an Inquiry by Sir William Macpherson of Cluny. London: The Stationery Office. (Cm 4262–I). Available at: https://www.gov.uk/government/publications/the-stephen-lawrence-inquiry (Accessed: 29 April 2025).

Makhoul Khoury, S., Cohen, A., Fabris, M.A. and Gur, A. (2025) 'Neglect of children with disabilities: A scoping review', *Children*, 12(3), p 386.

Mallick, K. (2023) *Testimony to the UK COVID-19 Inquiry*, Disability Rights UK.

Martin, R. (2019) *Witness statement of Sir Robert Martin*. 17 October. Abuse in Care Royal Commission of Inquiry. Available at: https://www.abuseincare.org.nz/__data/assets/pdf_file/0028/26947/witness-statement-of-sir-robert-martin-17-october-2019.pdf (Accessed: 2 November 2025).

Martin, S., Longo, F., Lomas, J. and Claxton, K. (2021) 'Causal impact of social care, public health and healthcare expenditure on mortality in England: Cross-sectional evidence for 2013/2014', *BMJ Open*, 11(10), e046417.

Mason, M. (1990) 'Internalized Oppression', in Reiser, R. and Mason, M. (eds) *Disability Equality in Education*, London: ILEA. Available at: https://disability-studies.leeds.ac.uk/wp-content/uploads/sites/40/library/Mason-Michelene-mason.pdf (Accessed: 5 April 2025).

Maung, H.H. (2023) 'Externalist argument against medical assistance in dying for psychiatric illness', *Journal of Medical Ethics*, 49(8), pp 553–557.

Mbembe, A. (2003) 'Necropolitics', *Public Culture*, 15(1), pp 11–40.

McCarthy, M. (2017) '"What kind of abuse is him spitting in my food?": Reflections on the similarities between disability hate crime, so-called 'mate'crime and domestic violence against women with intellectual disabilities', *Disability & Society*, 32(4), pp 595–600.

McCarthy, M., Hunt, S. and Milne-Skillman, K. (2017) 'I know it was every week, but I can't be sure if it was every day: Domestic violence and women with learning disabilities', *Journal of Applied Research in Intellectual Disabilities*, 30(2), pp 269–282.

McCausland, R. and Dowse, L. (2022) 'From "at risk" to "a risk": The criminalisation of young people with cognitive disability in residential care', *Incarceration*, 3(1), pp 1–14.

McKinney, J.C. (1966) *Constructive Typology and Social Theory*, New York: Appleton-Century-Crofts.

McRuer, R. (2006) *Crip Theory: Cultural Signs of Queerness and Disability*, New York: New York University Press.

Meekosha, H. (2011) 'Decolonising disability: Thinking through the Global South', *Disability & Society*, 26(6), pp 667–682.

Mental Capacity Act 2005. Available at: https://www.legislation.gov.uk/ukpga/2005/9/contents/enacted (Accessed: 23 April 2025).

Milton, D. (2012) 'On the ontological status of autism: The "double empathy problem"', *Disability & Society*, 27(6), pp 883–887.

Mingus, M. (2017) 'Access intimacy: The missing link', *Leaving Evidence*. Available at: https://leavingevidence.wordpress.com/2011/05/05/access-intimacy-the-missing-link/

Ministry of the Solicitor General, Office of the Chief Coroner (2024) *MAiD Death Review Committee Report 2024–3: Navigating Vulnerability in Non-Reasonably Foreseeable Natural Deaths*, Ontario: Ministry of the Solicitor General. Available at: https://www.ontario.ca/document/maid-death-review-committee-report-2024-3 (Accessed: 27 April 2025).

Minkowitz, T. (2007) 'The United Nations Convention on the Rights of Persons with Disabilities and the right to be free from nonconsensual psychiatric interventions', *Syracuse Journal of International Law and Commerce*, 34(2), pp 405–428.

Mitchell, D. and Snyder, S. (2015) *The Biopolitics of Disability: Neoliberalism, Ablenationalism, and Peripheral Embodiment*, Ann Arbor: University of Michigan Press.

Montanari Vergallo, G., Varone, M.C. and Del Rio, A. (2021) 'COVID-19: When health care resources run short, how to pick who should (not) get treated?', *Acta Biomedica*, 92(4), e2021372.

Mostert, M.P. (2002) 'Useless eaters: Disability as genocidal marker in Nazi Germany', *The Journal of Special Education*, 36(3), pp 157–170.

Mushimiyimana, G. (2018) 'Women and girls with disabilities' issues in the light of grassroots experience', in Humanity & Inclusion (ed) *Gender and disability intersectionality in practice: Women and girls with disabilities addressing discrimination and violence in Africa*, Lyon: Humanity & Inclusion, p 5.

National Council on Disability (2020) *Statement on the Death of Michael Hickson*. Available at: https://www.ncd.gov/2020/07/02/ncd-chairman-statement-on-death-of-michael-hickson/ (Accessed: 27 April 2025).

National Council on Disability (2021) *COVID-19 and People with Disabilities*. Available at: https://www.ncd.gov/assets/uploads/reports/2021/ncd-2021-progress-report-covid-19.pdf (Accessed: 27 April 2025).

Ne'eman, A. (2020) '"I Will Not Apologize for My Needs": Even in a Pandemic, Doctors Should Not Abandon the Principle of Nondiscrimination', *The New York Times*, 23 March 2020.

Nixon, R. (2011) *Slow Violence and the Environmentalism of the Poor*, Cambridge, MA: Harvard University Press.

Not Dead Yet (n.d.) *Disability rights opposition to assisted suicide and euthanasia*.

Occupy Mental Health Project (2012) *Mindful occupation: rising up without burning out*, Richmond, VA: RVA Icarus. Available at: https://mindfuloccupation.org/files/booklet/mindful_occupation_singles_latest.pdf (Accessed: 28 April 2025).

O'Dell, L., Bertilsdotter Rosqvist, H., Ortega, F., Brownlow, C. and Orsini, M. (2016) 'Critical autism studies: Exploring epistemic dialogues and intersections, challenging dominant understandings of autism', *Disability & Society*, 31(2), pp 166–179.

Office for National Statistics (ONS) (2022) *Updated Estimates of Coronavirus (COVID-19) Related Deaths by Disability Status, England: 24 January 2020 to 9 March 2022*. Available at: https://www.ons.gov.uk/peoplepopulationandcommunity/birthsdeathsandmarriages/deaths/articles/coronaviruscovid19relateddeathsbydisabilitystatusenglandandwales/24january2020to9march2022 (Accessed: 27 April 2025).

Office of the United Nations High Commissioner for Human Rights (2020) *COVID-19 and the Rights of Persons with Disabilities: Guidance*, Geneva: United Nations. Available at: https://www.ohchr.org/en/documents/tools-and-resources/covid-19-and-rights-persons-disabilities-guidance (Accessed: 27 April 2025).

O'Sullivan, C., and McNamara, D. (2021) 'The "necessity" of austerity and its relationship with the UN Convention on the Rights of Persons with Disabilities: A case study of Ireland and the United Kingdom', *Human Rights Law Review*, 21(1), pp 157–185.

O'Sullivan, J. (2024) *Witness Statement provided by Jackie O'Sullivan on behalf of the Royal Mencap Society, 22 May 2024*. Module 3 evidence: INQ000479878. London: UK Covid-19 Inquiry. Available at: https://www.covid19.public-inquiry.uk/documents/inq000479878-witness-statement-provided-by-jackie-osullivan-on-behalf-of-the-royal-mencap-society-dated-22-05-2024/ (Accessed: 3 November 2025).

Oliver, M. (1990) *The Politics of Disablement*, London: Macmillan.

Ouellette, A. (2017) 'Barriers to physician aid in dying for people with disabilities', *Laws*, 6(4), 23.

Oregon Health Authority (2023) 'Death with Dignity Act – Frequently Asked Questions', *Oregon.gov*. Available at: https://www.oregon.gov/oha/ph/providerpartnerresources/evaluationresearch/deathwithdignityact/pages/faqs.aspx (Accessed: 17 September 2025).

Parrock, J. (2020) 'European Disabled Groups Worry about Threat to Independent Living Amid COVID-19', *Euronews*, 14 April. Available at: https://www.euronews.com/my-europe/2020/04/14/european-disabled-groups-worry-about-threat-to-independent-living-amid-covid-19 (Accessed: 27 April 2025).

Perlin, M.L. (2012) *International Human Rights and Mental Disability Law: When the Silenced are Heard*, Oxford: Oxford University Press.

Piepzna-Samarasinha, L.L. (2018) *Care Work: Dreaming Disability Justice*, Vancouver: Arsenal Pulp Press.

Piepzna-Samarasinha, L.L. (2021) 'How Disabled Mutual Aid Is Different Than Abled Mutual Aid', *Disability Visibility Project*, 3 October. Available at: https://disabilityvisibilityproject.com/2021/10/03/how-disabled-mutual-aid-is-different-than-abled-mutual-aid/ (Accessed: 27 April 2025).

Prince, M.J. (2016) *Struggling for Social Citizenship: Disabled Canadians, Income Security, and Prime Ministerial Eras*, Montreal: McGill-Queen's University Press.

Pring, J. (2025) 'Government proposes scrapping key benefits safeguard despite suicide risk', *Disability News Service*, 28 February. Available at: https://www.disabilitynewsservice.com/government-proposes-scrapping-key-benefits-safeguard-despite-suicide-risk/ (Accessed: 28 February 2025).

Puar, J.K. (2017) *The Right to Maim: Debility, Capacity, Disability*. Durham: Duke University Press.

Quarmby, K. (2011) *Scapegoat: Why We are Failing Disabled People*. London: Portobello Books.

Raus, K. (2016) 'The extension of Belgium's euthanasia law to include competent minors', *Journal of Bioethical Inquiry*, 13(2), pp 305–315.

Reed, P. (2024) 'Discrimination against the dying', *Journal of Medical Ethics*, 50, pp 108–114.

Reeve, D. (2012) 'Psycho-emotional disablism: The missing link?', in Watson, N., Roulstone, A. and Thomas, C. (eds) *Routledge Handbook of Disability Studies*, London: Routledge, pp 78–92.

Reynolds, J.M., Guidry-Grimes, L. and Savin, K. (2021) 'Against personal ventilator reallocation', *Cambridge Quarterly of Healthcare Ethics*, 30(2), pp 272–284.

Riley, A., Daruwalla, N., Kanougiya, S., Gupta, A., Wickenden, M. and Osrin, D. (2022) 'Intimate partner violence against women with disability and associated mental health concerns: A cross-sectional survey in Mumbai, India', *BMJ Open*, 12(4), e056475.

Roff, C. and Cook-Cottone, C. (2024) 'Assisted death in eating disorders: A systematic review of cases and clinical rationales', *Frontiers in Psychology*, 15, 1431771.

Rosenthal, E. (2021) 'Residential Care Controversy: The promise of the UN Convention on the Rights of Persons with Disabilities to protect all children', *International Journal of Disability and Social Justice*, 1(1), pp 95–117.

Rossiter, K. and Rinaldi, J. (2018) *Institutional Violence and Disability: Punishing Conditions*, London: Routledge.

Roulstone, A., Thomas, P. and Balderston, S. (2011) 'Between hate and vulnerability: Unpacking the British criminal justice system's construction of disablist hate crime', *Disability & Society*, 26(3), pp 351–364.

Ryan, F. (2019) *Crippled: Austerity and the Demonization of Disabled People*, London: Verso.

Ryan, S. (2017) *Justice for Laughing Boy: Connor Sparrowhawk – A Death by Indifference*, London: Jessica Kingsley Publishers.

Sallnow, L., Smith, R., Ahmedzai, S.H., Bhadelia, A., Chamberlain, C., Cong, Y., et al (2025) 'Report of the Lancet Commission on the value of death: Bringing death back into life', *The Lancet*, 405(10321), pp 102–127.

Schalk, S. (2018) *Bodyminds Reimagined: (Dis)ability, Race, and Gender in Black Women's Speculative Fiction*, Durham: Duke University Press.

Scobie, S., Hutchings, R., Davies, M., Kumpunen, S. and Reed, S. (2025) *Assisted Dying in Practice: International Experiences and Implications for Health and Social Care*, London: Nuffield Trust.

Series, L. (2022) *Deprivation of Liberty in the Shadows of the Institution*, Bristol: Bristol University Press.

Shakespeare, T. (2013) *Disability Rights and Wrongs Revisited* (2nd edn), London: Routledge.

Shakespeare, T. (2022) 'Written evidence submitted by Tom Shakespeare (ADY0021)', *UK Parliament Assisted Dying Inquiry*. Available at: https://www.parliament.uk/ (Accessed: 17 September 2025).

Shannon, P., Wilson, N.J. and Blythe, S. (2023) 'Out-of-home care for children with intellectual and developmental disabilities: A scoping review', *Hindawi Health & Social Care in the Community*, 2023, Article ID 2422367, 20 pages.

Shapira, S. and Granek, L. (2019) 'Negotiating psychiatric cisgenderism–ableism in the transgender–autism nexus', *Feminism & Psychology*, 29(4), pp 494–513.

Sharpe, C. (2016) *In the Wake: On Blackness and Being*, Durham, NC: Duke University Press.

Shelton, T. and Yang, S. (2020) 'Death of disabled teen after father quarantined with coronavirus in China sees two officials sacked', *ABC News*. 4 February. Available at: https://www.abc.net.au/news/2020-02-04/coronavirus-disabled-boy-dies-in-china-after-father-quarantined/11927180 (Accessed: 30 April 2025).

Shildrick, M. (2002) *Embodying the Monster: Encounters with the Vulnerable Self*, London: SAGE.

Shildrick, M. (2012) *Dangerous Discourses of Disability, Subjectivity and Sexuality*, Basingstoke: Palgrave Macmillan.

SIAARTI (2020) *Clinical Ethics Recommendations for the Allocation of Intensive Care Treatments in Exceptional, Resource-Limited Circumstances*, Rome: Italian Society of Anesthesia, Analgesia, Resuscitation and Intensive Care.

Sidanius, J. and Pratto, F. (1999) *Social Dominance: An Intergroup Theory of Social Hierarchy and Oppression*, Cambridge: Cambridge University Press.

Sin, C.H., Hedges, A., Cook, C., Mguni, N. and Comber, N. (2009) *Disabled People's Experiences of Targeted Violence and Hostility*, Manchester: Equality and Human Rights Commission.

Sin, C.H., Sheikh, S. and Khanna, M. (2012) 'Police readiness for tackling hate crime against people with learning disabilities – areas for improvement and examples of good practice', *Safer Communities*, 11(3), pp 145–153.

Šiška, J. and Beadle-Brown, J. (2023) 'Progress on deinstitutionalisation and the development of community living for persons with disabilities in Europe: Are we nearly there?', *Disability & Society*, 38(8), pp 1476–1495.

Stainton, T. (2023) 'Assisted life before assisted death: Disability discomfort regarding MAID', in Kotalik, J. and Shannon, D.W. (eds) *Medical assistance in dying (MAID) in Canada*, Cham: Springer, pp 309–323.

Stalker, K. and McArthur, K. (2012) 'Child abuse, child protection and disabled children: A review of recent research', *Child Abuse Review*, 21(1), pp 24–40.

St. Pierre, J. (2015) 'Distending straight-masculine time: A phenomenology of the disabled speaking body', *Hypatia*, 30(1), pp 49–65.

Steele, L. (2014) 'Disability, abnormality and criminal law: Sterilisation as lawful and "good" violence', *Griffith Law Review*, 23(3), pp 467–497.

Steele, L. (2020) *Disability, criminal justice and law: Reconsidering court diversion*, London: Routledge.

Stringer, M. (2023) *Witness Statement on Behalf of the Disability Charities Consortium. UK COVID-19 Inquiry, Module 3*, INQ000235594.

Sudnow, D. (1967) *Passing On: The Social Organization of Dying*, Englewood Cliffs, NJ: Prentice-Hall.

Sue, D.W. and Spanierman, L.B. (2020) *Microaggressions in Everyday Life* (2nd edn), Hoboken, NJ: Wiley.

Sue, D.W., Capodilupo, C.M., Torino, G.C., Bucceri, J.M., Holder, A.M.B., Nadal, K.L. and Esquilin, M. (2007) 'Racial microaggressions in everyday life: Implications for clinical practice', *American Psychologist*, 62(4), pp 271–286.

Sumner, L.W. (2011) *Assisted Death: A Study in Ethics and Law*, Oxford: Oxford University Press.

Taylor, P., Corteen, K., Ogden, C. and Morley, S. (2012) '"Standing by": Disability hate crime and the police in England', *Criminal Justice Matters*, 87(1), pp 46–47.

The Arc, Autistic Self Advocacy Network, Bazelon Center for Mental Health Law and Disability Rights Texas (2025) *Amicus Brief in Hickson v. St. David's Healthcare Partnership*. Available at: https://thearc.org/wp-content/uploads/2025/04/Hickson-Amicus-Brief.pdf (Accessed: 28 April 2025).

Thomas, C. (2007) *Sociologies of Disability and Illness: Contested Ideas in Disability Studies and Medical Sociology*, Basingstoke: Palgrave Macmillan.

Thorneycroft, R. (2020) 'Crip theory and Mad Studies: Intersections and points of departure', *Canadian Journal of Disability Studies*, 9(1), pp 91–122.

Timmermans, S. and Sudnow, D. (1998) 'Social death as self-fulfilling prophecy: David Sudnow's "passing on" revisited', *The Sociological Quarterly*, 39(3), pp 453–472.

Titchkosky, T. (2003) *Disability, Self, and Society*, Toronto: University of Toronto Press.

Toman, N. (2023) *Witness Statement on Behalf of Disability Action Northern Ireland. UK COVID-19 Inquiry, Module 3*, INQ000348704.

Tracey, R (on the Application of) v Cambridge University Hospitals NHS Foundation Trust & Ors [2014] EWCA Civ 822.

Tremain, S. (ed) (2005) *Foucault and the Government of Disability*, Ann Arbor: University of Michigan Press.

Tremain, S. (ed) (2015) *Foucault and the Government of Disability* (2nd edn), Ann Arbor: University of Michigan Press.

Tremain, S. (2017) *Foucault and Feminist Philosophy of Disability*, Ann Arbor: University of Michigan Press.

Tremain, S. (2019) 'Feminist philosophy of disability: A genealogical intervention', *The Southern Journal of Philosophy*, 57(1), pp 132–158.

UK COVID-19 Inquiry (2024) *Module 1 Report: The Resilience and Preparedness of the United Kingdom*. Available at: https://covid19.public-inquiry.uk/publications/module-1-report/ (Accessed: 25 April 2025).

UKHSA (2025) 'Who's eligible for the 2025 COVID-19 vaccine or autumn booster?', *UKHSA Blog*, 26 June. Available at: https://ukhsa.blog.gov.uk/2025/06/26/whos-eligible-for-the-2025-covid-19-vaccine-or-autumn-booster/ (Accessed: 17 September 2025).

UN Press Release (2020) *Secretary-General Policy Brief on Persons with Disabilities and COVID-19*, New York: United Nations.

UNICEF (2025) *Situation Analysis of Children and Adolescents in Kazakhstan: Summary Report. UNICEF Kazakhstan*. Available at: https://www.unicef.org/kazakhstan/en/media/13626/file/2025%20SitAn_Summary%20report_final_Eng%20(21%20Sept%202025).pdf.pdf.pdf.pdf) (Accessed: 20 November 2025).

United Nations Committee on the Rights of Persons with Disabilities (2017) *Concluding observations on the combined second and third periodic reports of Argentina (CRPD/C/ARG/CO/2–3)*, Geneva: United Nations, p 13.

United Nations Committee on the Rights of Persons with Disabilities (2015) *Concluding observations on the combined second and third periodic reports of Germany (CRPD/C/DEU/CO/2–3)*, Geneva: United Nations, pp 6, 14.

United Nations Committee on the Rights of Persons with Disabilities (2017) *Concluding observations on the initial report of Togo (CRPD/C/TGO/CO/1)*, Geneva: United Nations, p 6.

United Nations Committee on the Rights of Persons with Disabilities (2017) *Concluding observations on the initial report of Mauritania (CRPD/C/MRT/CO/1)*, Geneva: United Nations, para. 19.

United Nations Committee on the Rights of Persons with Disabilities (2021) *Concluding observations on the combined second and third periodic reports of Mongolia (CRPD/C/MNG/CO/2–3)*, Geneva: United Nations, para. 19.

United Nations Committee on the Rights of Persons with Disabilities (2022) *Concluding observations on the initial report of Georgia (CRPD/C/GEO/CO/1)*, Geneva: United Nations, para. 21.

United Nations Committee on the Rights of Persons with Disabilities (2022) *Concluding observations on the initial report of Israel (CRPD/C/ISR/CO/1)*, Geneva: United Nations, para. 21.

United Nations Committee on the Rights of Persons with Disabilities (2022) *Concluding observations on the combined second and third periodic reports of Canada (CRPD/C/CAN/CO/2–3)*, Geneva: United Nations, para. 10.

United Nations Committee on the Rights of Persons with Disabilities (2022) *Concluding observations on the combined first and second periodic reports of Malawi (CRPD/C/MWI/CO/1–2)*, Geneva: United Nations, para. 21(b).

United Nations Committee on the Rights of Persons with Disabilities (2023) *Concluding observations on the combined second and third periodic reports of Sweden (CRPD/C/SWE/CO/2–3)*, Geneva: United Nations, para. 41(a).

United Nations Committee on the Rights of Persons with Disabilities (2022) *Concluding observations on the initial report of Sweden (CRPD/C/SWE/CO/1)*, Geneva: United Nations. Available at: https://docstore.ohchr.org/SelfServices/FilesHandler.ashx?enc=6QkG1d%2FPPRiCAqhKb7yhsoAqHRnqPrUhJ%2F9GpT7G%2FHVKS%2BrN%2F1xUC%2BPgFnVT1cJmgCruhJfyDvLdyQ7dcNIxqRb%2BRBGkKmY2X5lHyB%2BTZw%2FpQHxS%2FDnr6C7SrfmA (Accessed: 15 April 2025).

United Nations Office for Disaster Risk Reduction (UNDRR) (2015) *Sendai Framework for Disaster Risk Reduction 2015–2030*, Geneva: UNDRR. Available at: https://www.undrr.org/publication/sendai-framework-disaster-risk-reduction-2015-2030 (Accessed: 17 April 2025).

United Nations (1966) *International Covenant on Economic, Social and Cultural Rights (ICESCR)*, New York: United Nations. Available at: https://www.ohchr.org/en/instruments-mechanisms/instruments/international-covenant-economic-social-and-cultural-rights (Accessed: 17 April 2025).

United Nations (1979) *Convention on the Elimination of All Forms of Discrimination Against Women (CEDAW)*, New York: United Nations. Available at: https://www.ohchr.org/en/instruments-mechanisms/instruments/convention-elimination-all-forms-discrimination-against-women (Accessed: 17 April 2025).

United Nations Department of Economic and Social Affairs (2024) *The Sustainable Development Goals Report 2024*, New York: United Nations. Available at: https://unstats.un.org/sdgs/report/2024/ (Accessed: 23 April 2025).

United Nations (1984) *Convention Against Torture and Other Cruel, Inhuman or Degrading Treatment or Punishment (CAT)*, New York: United Nations. Available at: https://www.ohchr.org/en/instruments-mechanisms/instruments/convention-against-torture-and-other-cruel-inhuman-or-degrading (Accessed: 17 April 2025).

United Nations (1989) *Convention on the Rights of the Child (CRC)*, New York: United Nations. Available at: https://www.ohchr.org/en/instruments-mechanisms/instruments/convention-rights-child (Accessed: 17 April 2025).

United Nations (2006) *Convention on the Rights of Persons with Disabilities (CRPD)*, New York: United Nations. Available at: https://www.un.org/development/desa/disabilities/convention-on-the-rights-of-persons-with-disabilities.html (Accessed: 17 April 2025).

Verita (2014) *Independent Investigation into the Death of CS*, London: Verita.

Verita (2015) *Independent Review Into Issues That May Have Contributed to the Preventable Death of Connor Sparrowhawk. NHS England South Region and Oxfordshire Safeguarding Adults Board.* Available at: https://www.england.nhs.uk/wp-content/uploads/2015/10/indpndnt-rev-connor-sparrowhawk.pdf (Accessed: 20 November 2025).

Walach, V. and Petruželka, B. (2024) 'Violence and disablist hate crime against people with intellectual disabilities: Czech NGOs and service providers' experiences', *Disability & Society*, 39(12), pp 3164–3189.

Walby, S. (2013) 'Violence and society: Introduction to an emerging field of sociology', *Current Sociology*, 61(2), pp 95–111.

Walby, S., Towers, J., Balderston, S., Corradi, C., Francis, B., Heiskanen, M., Helweg-Larsen, K., et al (2017) *The Concept and Measurement of Violence against Women and Men*, Bristol: Policy Press.

Walter, B., Chung, D., Waters, R. and Watts, L. (2024) 'Exploring lived experience of family and domestic violence against women with disability: A scoping review', *Trauma, Violence, & Abuse*, 25(3), pp 1925–1937.

Warner, N. (2023) 'DNR Orders, Disability & the Right to Decide', *Counsel Magazine*, 12 June. Available at: https://www.counselmagazine.co.uk/articles/dnr-orders-disability-the-right-to-decide (Accessed: 17 April 2025).

Watson, N. and Shakespeare, T. (2023) *Expert Report on Disability and Structural Inequalities, submitted to the UK COVID-19 Inquiry.*

Wei, H.-S., Chang, H.-H. and Chen, J.-K. (2016) 'Bullying and victimisation among Taiwanese students in special schools', *International Journal of Disability, Development and Education*, 63(2), pp 246–259.

Wilson, B. (2021) 'Crisis standards of care may discriminate against patients with disabilities', *The Regulatory Review*, 1 November. Available at: https://www.theregreview.org/2021/11/01/wilson-crisis-standards-of-care-may-discriminate-against-patients-with-disabilities/ (Accessed: 28 April 2025).

Winch, R.F. (1947) 'Heuristic and empirical typologies: A job for factor analysis', *American Sociological Review*, 12(1), pp 68–75.

Winspear v City Hospitals Sunderland NHS Foundation Trust [2015] EWHC 3250 (QB).

Wissink, I.B., van Vugt, E., Moonen, X., Stams, G.-J.J.M. and Hendriks, J. (2015) 'Sexual abuse involving children with an intellectual disability: A narrative review', *Research in Developmental Disabilities*, 36, pp 20–35.

Wissink, I.B., van Vugt, E.S., Smits, I.A.M., Moonen, X.M.H. and Stams, G.J.J.M. (2018) 'Reports of sexual abuse of children in state care: A comparison between children with and without intellectual disability', *Journal of Intellectual & Developmental Disability*, 43(2), pp 152–163.

Wolbring, G. (2008) 'The politics of ableism', *Development*, 51(2), pp 252–258.

Wolbring, G. (2012) 'Expanding ableism: Taking down the ghettoization of impact of disability studies scholars', *Societies*, 2(3), pp 75–83.

Wolfensberger, W. (1975) 'The Origin and Nature of Our Institutional Models', in Kugel, R.B. and Wolfensberger, W. (eds) *Changing Patterns in Residential Services for the Mentally Retarded*, Washington, DC: President's Panel on Mental Retardation, pp 59–171.

Woods, R., Milton, D., Arnold, L. and Graby, S. (2018) 'Redefining critical autism studies: A more inclusive interpretation', *Disability & Society*, 33(6), pp 974–979.

World Federation of Right to Die Societies (2021) 'Colombian court reduced euthanasia criteria', *World Federation of Right to Die Societies*, 26 July. Available at: https://wfrtds.org/colombian-court-reduced-euthanasia-criteria/ (Accessed: 27 April 2025).

World Health Organization (2002) *World report on violence and health*, Geneva: World Health Organization.

World Health Organization (2015) *WHO global disability action plan 2014–2021: better health for all people with disability*, Geneva: World Health Organization.

World Health Organization (2022) *Global report on health equity for persons with disabilities*, Geneva: World Health Organization.

X and Others v Hungary (Application no. 35943/18, European Court of Human Rights, 2023).

Yergeau, M. (2018) *Authoring Autism: On Rhetoric and Neurological Queerness*, Durham, NC: Duke University Press.

Young, K.G. (2019) *Waiting for rights: progressive realization and lost time.* Boston College Law School, Legal Studies Research Paper Series No. 509. Available at: https://ssrn.com/abstract=3428718 (Accessed: 28 April 2025).

Žižek, S. (2008) *Violence: Six Sideways Reflections*, London: Profile.

Index

References to tables appear in **bold** type.

A

ableist economies of doubt 33
Ableist Microaggression Scale 57–58
ablenationalism 38
abolition 81, 83
abuse
  of children 54–55, 64–65
  discretionary abuse 9
  domestic abuse, among disabled women 52–53
  in institutional settings 25, 29, 77–78
  microaggressions 59
  sexual abuse 54–55
access practices, collective 45
active euthanasia 89, 94, 95, 97
affect theory 51
Agamben, G. 35
Ahmed, S. 10
alternative care 18, 64
Annamma, S.A. 39
anthropemic strategies 71
anticipatory corpse 92, 98
antisocial behaviour, harassment as 56, 63
assisted dying
  as acts of commission 94–95
  as acts of omission 95–96
  in Belgium 93, 94, 97
  in Canada (MAID) 92–93, 94, 96–97
  in Colombia 93, 96
  conceptual framework 89–91
  expansion of eligibility 90–91, 92–94, 100
  framing as choice and autonomy 91, 100
  in Netherlands 94
  in Oregon 90
  and quality of life assessments 94, 97
  resistance to 98–100
  and suffering 93, 94–95, 98–99
  and terminalism 89–91, 94
Australia 76, 82, 116
austerity policies 2, 16, 38
autism 17, 33, 72, 94, 112
autonomy 9, 23–24, 44, 71, 82, 91, 97–98, 99–100, 101, 114

B

Baroness Hallett DBE, Rt Hon. 110
Bauman, Z. 25, 27, 36, 39, 71, 76, 110
Beckett, A.E. 10, 32, 81
Belgium 93, 94, 97, 111
Ben-Moshe, L. 71, 73, 80, 81, 83, 110
bioethics 44, 89, 91, 93
biopower 25, 32, 91–92, 112
Bishop, J. 92, 94, 98
Borg, K. 32
Bulgaria 81
Burch, L. 51, 65
bureaucratic rationality 76, 113
bureaucratic violence 27
burden-based motivations 90
Burstow, B. 17
Butler, J. 25, 40

C

Campbell, F.K. 30, 31, 32
Canada 75, 76, 82, 83, 92, 96–97
  Gauthier, Christine, case 96
  Health Canada reports 92
  Medical Assistance in Dying (MAID) 92, 96–97
  removal of 'reasonably foreseeable death' 92, 97
  Foley, Roger, case 96
capacity of discernment 97
capitalism 37–38
carceral archipelago/logics 23, 110
  concept of 71, 72–73, 76
  mutation through deinstitutionalisation 80–81
  post-carceral landscape 80–81, 84–85
care collectives, mutual aid and 45
care homes 23, 77, 109
  abuse in care settings 55
  as death traps 110
  deaths representing percentage of COVID deaths 110
  in Sweden 107–108
  visible as tragedy, invisible as preventable neglect 114
Care Quality Commission (CQC) 109
Castrodale, M.A. 33
CEDAW (Convention on the Elimination of All Forms of Discrimination Against Women) **13**, 15
chemical restraint 77
Cheng, Yan, case 108, 111
child protection systems 8, 55, 64–65
children, disabled
  abuse and neglect of 54–55

CRC (UN Convention on the Rights of the Child) **13**, 18
cultural devaluation of 54–55
disposability of 76
over-representation in institutionalisation 75
power dynamics and 54
resistance by 74, 82–83
sexual abuse of 54, 55
Children's Commissioner (UK) 77
China 108
Christian, J.M. 24, 26, 105
Clare, Eli 39
classification and differentiation, in *dispositif* 38–39, 74–76
Clinical Frailty Score 107
Clough, B. 16
coercion 41, 71, 97, 99
collateral damage framing 106
collective access practices 45
Colleran, M. 97
Colombia 93, 96
commission (violence by) 6, **20**, **21**, 22, 26, 84, 101, 105
in assisted dying contexts 94–95
COVID-19 pandemic 113–114
definition 6
in disability contexts 7–8
hate crimes as 7, 51
in institutional settings 73–74, 77–78
microaggressions as 56–57, 59–60
restraint as 14, 25, 77
commission by omission (violence by) 6, **21**, 22, 84, 101
in assisted dying contexts 96–97
COVID-19 pandemic 26, 105, 113–114
defined 8
DNAR orders 8, 10, 26, 78–79
domestic violence context 53
in institutional settings 73–74, 78–79
medical dismissal as 8, 14
microaggressions as 57, 59–60
professional discretion 55
purposeful neglect 8
theoretical development 26
triage decisions as 22
in violence against children 55
in violence against women 53
community abandonment 111
complex personhood 74, 82–83, 85
compulsory able-bodiedness 34, 54
confinement 17, 46, 47, 67, 70–72, 83–85, 100–101
acts of commission 77–78
acts of omission 78
acts of commission by omission 78–79
acts of omission by commission 79–80
beyond physical architecture 70
COVID-19 pandemic and 110
deinstitutionalisation 80–81
as denial of personhood 71
production of 74–76
resistance and complex personhood 82–83
soft confinement 76
theorising 72–74
Cook-Cottone, C. 93
cost-benefit analyses 80, 40, 113
counter-conduct 32, 37, 82
COVID-19 Disability Rights Monitor 116
COVID-19 pandemic 97, 101
as acceleration of ableist systems 105, 112
acts of commission 113
acts of omission 113
commission by omission during 26, 105, 113–114
community abandonment 111–112
confinements and 110
as critical juncture 105
disabled deaths statistics 106, 108
global catastrophe 106–108
lines of force 115
lines of subjectivation 115
lines of utterance 114–115
lines of visibility 114
mutual aid networks during 46, 115–116, 117
necropolitics of response 112–113
omission by commission during 114
in UK 108–110
resistance within 115–116
as revelatory moment 105, 112, 116–118
criminal justice systems 9, 51–52, 63
Critical Autism Studies 30, 33
crip technoscience 46
crip theory 34
crip time 35
CRPD (UN Convention on the Rights of Persons with Disabilities) 1, **12**, 16, 99
Article 4(3) 99
Article 8 (awareness- raising) 63
Article 10 (right to life) 11, 99
Article 12 (equal recognition before law) 16, 99
Article 13 (access to justice) 63
Article 25 (right to health) 11, 99
Committee 15, 18, 27, 70, 80, 81, 99
Concluding Observations 19–23
General Comment No. 1 16
position on group homes 81
Čuković, Jasmina 83
Czech Republic 51

D

Davis, L.J. 32
deinstitutionalisation 70–71, 80–82

Deleuze, Gilles 34–37, 43, 45, 60, 82
deontological ethics 107, 108
Department for Work and Pensions 2
differential grievability 25, 85, 91, 101
disablism vs ableism 31
Disability Charities Consortium 108
Disability Rights Education and Defense Fund 116
Disability Rights International (DRI) 75–76, 78, 79–80, 81
Disability Studies 2, 72, 84
  ableism perspectives 33–34
  assisted dying debates within 89, 91
  foundations 23–24
  Foucauldian approaches in 32
DisCrit scholars 34, 39, 44
dispositif
  as analytical framework 35–37
  defined by Foucault 35, 36
  discursive and representational domain 43
  embodied and psycho-emotional domain 44
  four lines analysis *see* lines of force; lines of subjectivation; lines of utterance; lines of visibility
  heterogeneity, characterised by 36
  institutional and administrative domain 43
  intersectional and differential domain 44
  material and architectural domain 43
  normative and ethical domain 44
  processual nature, characterised by 36
  strategic function, characterised by 36
  strategic reversibility 116
dispositif of violence 17, 24, 28, 70, 72, 84–85, 89, 91, 94, 98–101, 105, 112, 122–123
  classification and differentiation 38–39, 74–76
  hate crimes and 51–52
  identity formation and subjectivation 40
  institutional continuity of 55–56
  knowledge production and expertise 39–40
  microaggressions and 56–62
  normalisation and correction 39
  resource allocation and distribution 40
  spatial and temporal organisation 39
  see also commission (violence by); commission by omission (violence by); omission (violence by); omission by commission (violence by)
dividing practices 74
DNAR (Do Not Attempt Resuscitation) orders 1, 8, 26
  blanket application 109
  inappropriate application 108–109, 113
  legal precedents (Tracey, Winspear cases) 109
  reframed as 'palliative appropriateness' 105, 114
  without consultation 109, 113
Doherty, A. 97
domestic violence, against disabled women 53–54
Dowler, L. 24, 26, 105

E

eating disorders 93
Ebben, H. 33
economic prioritisation 97–98
emergency planning failures 109–110
epistemic injustice, ableism operating through 33
epistemic resistance 116, 117
epistemic violence 17, 33, 75, 84
epilepsy 72, 75, 78
Erevelles, N. 44
European Network for Independent Living 110
European Union (EU) 17
euthanasia 93, 96
  active 89, 94, 95, 97
  passive 89, 97
  see also assisted dying
Euser, S. 55
everyday ableism 24
exception clauses in legal frameworks 15
expendability of disabled lives 105, 107, 115
externalism 98, 101

F

family advocacy and resistance 83, 85
family knowledge, devaluation of 72, 75, 83, 84
fast violence 26, 27
Feely, M. 34
Finegan, T. 90
Flynn, E. 54–55, 64
Foley, Roger, case 96
forced medication 17, 73
Foucault, Michel 5, 15, 25, 26, 32, 35, 36, 37, 42, 45, 51, 91–92, 116
  biopower 25, 91–92
  carceral archipelago 73
  dispositif, defined 35, 36
  dividing practices 74
  institutions 25
  microphysics of power 77
  power and resistance 82
  strategy without strategist 93
fragility, feelings of 111
Fritsch, K. 46
funding models 79–80, 85

G

Galgay, C.E. 57
García-Cuéllar, M.M. 52
Gauci, V. 34
Gauthier, Christine, case 96
gender and violence 34, 52–54, 63–64
Germany 77, 107
Giménez, César 111
Gleeson, B. 38
Goffman, E. 70
Goodley, D. 9–10, 38, 44, 111, 115, 116
Granek, L. 33
Greece 77
Grech, S. 10
grievability, differential 25, 85, 91, 101
Griffiths, M. 89, 123
group homes 18, 71, 81, 110
Grue, J. 91–92
Guattari, F. 34, 37, 45, 82
Guatemala 79–80
Gurbai, Sándor 15
Guterres, António 106

H

Hall, E. 56, 63
Hamraie, A. 46
Han, C. 90
hate crimes 9, 53, 66–67
  ableism and 51–52
  harassment as 56
  institutional failure and 63
  insufficient legal recognition of 18–19
  violence by commission 7, 26
hate relationships 52
hate/vulnerability binary 52, 63
Healy, J.C. 53
Health Canada 92
Helton, J.J. 54
Hickson, Michael, case 11, 14, 97, 116
Hollomotz, A. 23
Holness, W. 51
hospice funding deficiencies (UK) 97–98
Huggins, Richard 83
Hughes, B. 9
human rights
  CRPD *see* CRPD (UN Convention on the Rights of Persons with Disabilities)
  violations during COVID-19 105, 108–110
  frameworks 10–19, 27
  legal recognition of violence 10–19
Human Rights Watch (HRW) 75, 77–78, 80, 83
human waste 25, 27, 36, 39, 71, 76
Hutcheon, E.J. 40
hypervisibility/invisibility paradox 36, 61, 105, 112, 114

I

ICESCR (International Covenant on Economic, Social and Cultural Rights) **13**, 15
identity formation and subjectivation 40, 61
implementation obligations, vague 15–16
Inclusion London 109, 111, 116
independent living movements 70, 123
India 52, 75
indigenous youth 76, 82, 83
Indonesia 77
institutional abandonment 108, 111
institutional archipelago 73, 76, 80, 84
institutional deaths 105, 110, 114
institutional violence 43, 84
institutionalisation 23, 74, 75, 78, 81, 83, 95
  legal frameworks facilitating 80
  as normalisation and control 84
  over-representation of disabled children 75
  persistence despite reform 17, 70–71, 85
  statistics 70–71
institutions
  as death traps 110
  Foucault on 25
  institutional and administrative domain of *dispositif* 43
  institutional continuity of ableist *dispositif* 55–56
  see also deinstitutionalisation; reinstitutionalisation
intellectual and developmental disabilities (IDDs) 75
intellectual/learning disabilities, sexual abuse and 55
interdependence
  relationality and 98, 101
  universal 10
internalised ableism 31, 37, 40–43, 56–57, 61, 115
international frameworks, legal recognition of violence in 10–14, **12–13**
intimate violence against disabled women 53
irremediability 93, 98
Israel 75
Italy 107

J

Johnk, L. 33
Jorge, Alice 111
#Justice4LB campaign 81, 83, 84

K

Kafer, A. 35, 39
Kattari, S.K. 57, 58, 65

Kavanagh, A.M. 116
Kazakhstan 77, 80
Keller, R.M. 57
Kittay, E.F. 98
Kiwan, D. 106
knowledge production and expertise 39–40
Kubenz, V. 106

L

Labour government 2
Lashewicz, B. 40
law as violence 14–15
lawful violence 14, 23–24
Lawrence, Stephen (murder of) 51
learning disabilities 8, 9, 16, 26, 34, 51, 53, 54, 64, 66
  in Australian residential care 76, 82
  categorised as 'frail' 107
  confinement and 70, 71, 76, 79, 82
  COVID-19 pandemic and residential care 112
  DNAR orders 108–109
  lack of statutory framework (UK) 79
  sexual abuse and 55
  vulnerability to institutionalisation 71
legal challenges 83, 116
legal frameworks
  exception clauses in 15
  facilitating institutionalisation 80
  insufficient recognition of hate crimes 18–19
  lack of disaggregated data 17–18
  medicalisation of disability in 16–17
  normalisation of segregation in 18
  vague implementation obligations in 15–16
legal protections 19, 22, 99
legal recognition of violence, international frameworks 10–14, **12–13**
LeFrançois, B.A. 17
Lewis, Olaseni (death of) 14
LGBTQIA+ disabled people 34
lines of flight
  in ableism as *dispositif* 37, 44–46
  collective resistance as 45–46, 66, 116
  in institutional contexts 82–83
  mutual aid as 45–46, 115–116
lines of force
  assisted dying and terminalism 91, 93, 101
  confinements 72, 73, 76, 79, 81, 84
  COVID-19 pandemic 105, 115
  hate crimes 60–61
  in ableism as *dispositif* 37, 40, 41
  microaggressions and 61
  professional authority as 60, 76
lines of subjectivation
  in ableism as *dispositif* 37, 42, 46
  assisted dying and terminalism 91, 93–94, 101
  confinements 72, 73, 81, 84
  COVID-19 pandemic 105, 115
  hate crimes 56–57, 61
  internalised ableism and 40–43
  microaggressions and 57, 61
lines of utterance
  in ableism as *dispositif* 36–37, 39, 41, 43–44
  in assisted dying discourse 91, 93, 101
  confinements 72, 73, 74–75, 79, 81, 84
  COVID-19 pandemic 105, 114–115
  hate crimes 52, 61
  microaggressions and 61
  professional knowledge and 39–40, 74–75
lines of visibility
  in ableism as *dispositif* 36, 39, 41, 43–44
  in assisted dying contexts 91, 93, 101
  confinements 72, 72, 73, 80–81, 84
  COVID-19 pandemic 105, 112, 114
  in domestic violence 53–54
  hate crimes 53–54, 61
  microaggressions and 61
litigation, political advocacy and 46
Löfvenberg, Latifa 107
Löfven, Stefan 107–108
long-term care facilities, and COVID-19 (US) 110
Longmore, P.K. 95, 99
Lord, J.E. 18
low- and middle-income countries 52, 106

M

Macdonald, S.J. 52
Macpherson Report (1999) 51
macroaggressions 105, 117
Mad Studies 30, 32–33, 71
Makhoul Koury, S. 54
managerialism in child protection systems 55, 64
marginalisation 1–2, 41, 76
Martin, S. 2
Martin, R. 70, 72, 74, 77, 78, 79, 80, 82, 83
Mason, M. 42
material and architectural domain (*dispositif*) 43
Maung, H.H. 93, 98
Mbembe, A. 91, 94, 112
McAfee, Larry, case 94–95
McCarthy, M. 53
McKinney, J.C. 6
McNamara, D. 16
Medical Assistance in Dying (MAID), Canada 92, 96–97

medical neglect 78
medical professional bodies 100
medicalisation
of death 94
of disability in legal frameworks 16–17, 27
Meekosha, H. 10
Mental Capacity Act 2005 (UK), Section 6 14
Mental Health Units (Use of Force) Act 2018 (UK) (Seni's Law) 14
microaggressions 56–62, 105, 117
as capillary level of *dispositif* 56–57
dispositif framework analysis 59–62
and everyday hostility 65
understanding and evidencing as violence 57–59
micro-invalidation/macro-invalidation 107
microphysics of power 77
Milton, D. 17
Minear, A. 44
Mingus, M. 45
Mitchell, D. 38
modernity and exclusion, Bauman on 25, 36, 39
monitoring, lack of disaggregated data for 17–18
Montanari Vergallo, G. 107
Mushimiyimana, G. 54, 64, 66
mutual aid networks 45, 46, 115–116, 117

N

National Council on Disability (US) 110
necropolitics 91, 112–113, 116
neglect 19, 24, 26, 45, 78, 105, 107, 114
institutional 5
medical neglect 78
permissive 26
purposeful 8
systematic 7, 51–52
see also abuse; omission (violence by)
neoliberalism 38, 44, 45, 91–92, 98, 101
Netherlands 54, 75, 94
New Zealand 70
Nixon, R. 16, 24, 26, 27, 38, 52, 62
normalisation
and correction 39
of segregation 18
normative and ethical domain (*dispositif*) 44
Norway 81
Not Dead Yet Campaign 89, 99

O

objective violence 24
O'Dell, L. 33
Office for National Statistics (UK) 106, 108
Office of the United Nations High Commissioner for Human Rights 110
Oliver, M. 38
omission (violence by) 4–5, 6, **20**, 22
absence of action 5
in assisted dying contexts 95–96
confinements 73–74, 78, 84
COVID-19 pandemic 105, 113
definition 6
in disability contexts 7–8
domestic violence context 53
microaggressions as 57, 59–60
neglect as 7–8, 78
theoretical development 26
in violence against children 55
omission by commission (violence by) **21**, 22, 27
in assisted dying contexts 97–98, 101
austerity measures as 16, 40
bureaucratic violence 27
COVID-19 pandemic 105, 114
defined 6, 8
in institutional settings 74, 79–80, 84
legal frameworks enabling 8, 14–18, 97–98
legislation and policy changes 8
microaggressions as 59–60
policy withdrawal as 6, 8, **20–21**
theoretical development 26–27
Oregon (USA) 90
O'Sullivan, C. 16
O'Sullivan, J. 109
Ouellette, A. 89
out-of-home care (OOHC) 55, 75

P

palliative care 95–96, 98, 99
parrhesiastic rhetoric 92
passive euthanasia 89, 97
personal assistance services 2, 27, 99, 111
Petruželka, B. 51
physical environments 39, 43
Pierce, C. 57
Piepzna-Samarasinha, L.L. 45, 115
Pilkington, Fiona (case of) 51–52, 56
police and policing 14, 26, 51–52, 56, 63, 67
Policy Brief on Persons with Disabilities and COVID-19 106
political advocacy and litigation 46
populism, right-wing 1–2
post-carceral landscape 80–81, 84–85
poverty 92, 93, 95, 106, 109
power
biopower 25, 32, 91–92, 112
disciplinary power 25
dynamics with children 54
Foucault on 45
microphysics of 77

power/knowledge 35
power relationship and violence 4–5
Taylor on 51
precarity 10, 25,40
proceduralism in child protection systems 55, 64
professional discretion 5, 55, 60, 114, 115
professional knowledge, critical role in *dispositif* 60, 72, 75, 81
progressive realisation 15–16
psychiatric cisgenderism-ableism 33
psychiatric survivor movement 71
psycho-emotional disablism 44, 62
psychosocial impairments 16, 93
Puar, J.K. 38

Q

quality-adjusted life years 40, 113
quality-of-life assessments 90, 93, 97, 107, 112, 114, 116
Queer Disability Studies 34

R

racism 24, 34
rational suicide 95
Raus, K. 97
Reed, P. 89–90
Reeve, D. 41, 42, 44, 62
reform 63
and abolition, distinction between 81
child protection and care 64–65
Labour government proposal 2
policy reform 9
structural reform 63
reinstitutionalisation 71
relationality and interdependence 98, 117
resistance
in assisted dying contexts 96, 98–100
by disabled children 74, 82–83
COVID-19 pandemic 115–116
epistemic resistance 116, 117
family advocacy 83
to hate crimes 65–66
to institutional violence 82–83
legal challenges 109, 116
to microaggressions 65
misinterpretation as pathology 82–83
mutual aid networks 115–116, 117
political advocacy 46
within crisis 115–116
resistance strategies
centring disabled voices 99, 101
challenges and constraints 99–100
collective organising 65–66, 99
externalist frameworks 101
human rights approaches 99, 101
practical interventions 99
relational ethics 98, 101
resource allocation 38, 44, 61, 74, 98
and distribution 40
frameworks 105, 113, 114–115, 117
maximum of available resources 15–16
restraint
chemical 77
in institutional settings 1, **12**, 14, 23, 25, 27, 77
legal provisions for 14–15
physical 14, 27, 77
Seni's Law 14
revelatory moment, pandemic as 105, 112, 116–117
rights expansion logic 97, 98
Rivlin, David, case 95
Roff, C. 93
Romania 110
Rosenthal, E. 18
Roulstone, A. 52
Royal Commission of Inquiry into Abuse in Care (New Zealand) 70
Royal Mencap Society 109
Russia 78
Russian invasion of Ukraine 76
Rwanda 54
Ryan, Sara 38, 40, 72, 81, 83

S

Sallnow, L. 96, 99
Schalk, S. 40
Scobie, S. 97–98
segregation, normalisation of 1, 18
self-advocacy movement 2, 66, 70, 116
Sendai Framework for Disaster Risk Reduction (2015–2030) **13**
Seni's Law (Mental Health Units Use of Force Act 2018) 14
Serbia 78, 83
Series, L. 73, 80, 84–85
sexism 24, 52–54, 63
sexual abuse of disabled children 54, 55, 81
Shakespeare, T. 34, 89, 109
Shapira, S. 33
Shildrick, M. 9
Sin, C.H. 51
slippery slope 92–94
slow violence 16, 24, 26, 27, 38, 52, 62, 78
slow/fast violence complex 26, 105
Snyder, S. 38
social care withdrawal 105, 114
social death 25, 26, 70, 85, 94, 112–113, 117
social vs biological solutions 95, 101
South Africa 51
Southern Health NHS Foundation Trust 72
Spain 75, 111

Sparrowhawk, Connor ('Laughing Boy')
  case analysis 72–73, 75, 78–79, 81, 84
  death circumstances 72, 78
  devaluation of family expertise 75
  dispositif analysis 72, 84
  #Justice4LB campaign 81, 83, 84
spatial and temporal organisation (*dispositif*) 39
St. Pierre, J. 35
Steele, L. 14, 23–24, 26
straight-masculine time 35, 39
strategic forgetting 117
strategic reversibility 116
strategy without strategist 93
Stringer, M. 108
structural inequalities 106, 109
structural violence 23, 44, 107
subjectivation
  identity formation and 40
  lines of *see* lines of subjectivation
subjective violence 24, 26
Sudnow, D. 25, 113
Sue, D.W. 57
suffering, and assisted dying 92–95, 98–99
support systems, collapse of 111
surveillance 17, 70, 73, 76, 81, 82, 84
Sweden 107–108

T

Taylor, P. 51, 63
'temporary safety suspensions' 105, 114
temporal dimension of violence 24, 27, 35
terminalism 89–90, 91
  acts of commission 94–95
  acts of omission 95–96
  commission by omission 96–97
  omission by commission 97–98
  resisting ableism as a *dispositif* of violence 98–100
thanatopolitics 91–92, 99, 100
theoretical framework, development of 24–25
Thomas, C. 44
Thorneycroft, R. 32–33
Timmermans, S. 113
Titchkosky, T. 32
total institution 70
Tracey, R (on the Application of) v Cambridge University Hospitals 109
'tragic but inevitable' framing 105, 114
transhumanised ableism 31
Tremain, S. 32
triage protocols 1, 26, 105, 107, 112, 114, 115, 117
Turning Point (charity) 107

U

UK Covid-19 Inquiry 108–110
Ukraine 75–76, 78
UN Convention Against Torture (CAT) **12**
UN Convention on the Rights of Persons with Disabilities *see* CRPD (UN Convention on the Rights of Persons with Disabilities)
UN Convention on the Rights of the Child (CRC) **13**, 18
UN Department of Economic and Social Affairs 17
United States 90, 110, 116
universal interdependence 10
utilitarian approaches 107, 108

V

vaccination eligibility, narrowing of 117
violence typology *see* commission (violence by); commission by omission (violence by); omission (violence by); omission by commission (violence by)
vulnerability 10, 52
'vulnerable populations' 105, 112, 114

W

Walach, V. 51
Walby, S. 5, 24, 44–45, 58
Walter, B. 53, 64
Warner, N. 109
wasted populations 25, 27, 39
Watson, N. 109
WHO (World Health Organization)
  definition of violence 4
  Global Disability Action Plan 2014–2021 **13**
Winspear v City Hospitals Sunderland NHS Foundation Trust 109
Winterbourne View scandal 9
Wissink, I.B. 54, 55
Wolbring, G. 30, 31–32
Wolfensberger, W. 70
women, disabled
  CEDAW **13**, 15
  compulsory able-bodiedness 54
  domestic violence against 53–54
  intimate violence against 53
  violence against 52–54
  see also gender
Work Capability Assessment, replacement of 2

Y

Yergeau, M. 17
Young, K.G. 16

Z

Žižek, S. 24, 26

Printed and bound by CPI Group (UK) Ltd, Croydon, CR0 4YY
15/09/2026
14962387-0003